BEST
WEIGHT

A PRACTICAL GUIDE TO OFFICE-BASED OBESITY MANAGEMENT

[by Yoni Freedhoff, MD, and Arya M. Sharma, MD, PhD]

Published by the Canadian Obesity Network - Réseau canadien en obésité (CON-RCO)

ISBN# 978-0-9865889-0-7

[ABOUT THE AUTHORS]

Dr. Yoni Freedhoff

Dr. Yoni Freedhoff, MD CCFP Dip ABBM, is the founder and Medical Director of the Bariatric Medical Institute in Ottawa, a multi-disciplinary behavioural weight-management program. Formally trained in family medicine, his practice has been exclusively dedicated to the treatment of overweight and obesity since 2004.

Dr. Freedhoff has been referred to as a "nutritional watchdog" by the *Canadian Medical Association Journal* and a national "obesity expert" by the Canadian Obesity Network. His advocacy efforts for improved public policies regarding nutrition and obesity have found him testifying in front of the Canadian House of Commons, giving press conferences with the Ontario Medical Association, commenting regularly in the national media, and freelancing for the *Canadian Medical Association Journal,* as well as being a sought-after lecturer.

Dr. Freedhoff is an active member of the Canadian Obesity Network, the Obesity Society, the American Society of Bariatric Physicians, the American Board of Bariatric Medicine, the Center for Science in the Public Interest, as well as the Canadian College of Family Physicians. He lectures regularly for the Department of Family Medicine at the University of Ottawa and explores issues pertinent to nutrition, obesity, public policy and advocacy in his daily blog, Weighty Matters, which is ranked among the world's top health blogs. It was voted the top Canadian health blog of 2008 by the Canadian Blog Awards: www.weightymatters.ca.

Dr. Arya M. Sharma

Dr. Arya M. Sharma is Professor of Medicine and Chairholder in Obesity Research and Management at the University of Alberta in Edmonton, Canada. He is also Medical Director of the Edmonton region interdisciplinary Weight Wise program and Scientific Director of the Canadian Obesity Network. He is currently the President of the Canadian Association of Bariatric Physicians and Surgeons.

His past appointments include positions as Professor of Medicine and Canada Research Chair (Tier 1) at McMaster University (2002–2007), Professor of Medicine at the Franz-Volhard Klinik – Charité, at Humboldt University in Berlin (2000–2002) and the Free University of Berlin (1994–2000). His research focuses on the evidence-based prevention and management of obesity and its complications.

Dr. Sharma is on the editorial boards of several international journals and has authored or co-authored more than 250 scientific articles. He has also lectured widely on the etiology and management of hypertension, obesity, and related cardiovascular disorders. Dr. Sharma is regularly featured as a medical expert in national and international television and print media including the CBC, CTV, *New York Times,* and MSNBC. Dr. Sharma maintains a widely read blog on which he regularly posts his ideas and thoughts on obesity prevention and management: www.drsharma.ca.

[ACKNOWLEDGEMENTS]

For our wonderful wives, children, and patients. – YF & AMS

The authors gratefully acknowledge the support of the Canadian Obesity Network in publishing this manuscript. Thanks to Patti Whitefoot-Bobier for design and typesetting, Brad Hussey for editing and project coordination, Green Ink for proofreading, and S. L. Strilesky for rights and permissions.

[INTRODUCTION]

We shouldn't have had to write this book.

Despite its status as the second most preventable cause of death in the developed world, sadly, very little time is spent on training physicians in the whys and wherefores of obesity treatment.

When we set out to open our weight-management practices, we were left to fend for ourselves in the development of our approaches. When we later met for the first time at the 2005 Annual Scientific Meeting of the Obesity Society, it quickly became evident that, despite our divergent backgrounds, our approaches and philosophies surrounding weight management were quite complementary and reflected the overlapping circles of specialist tertiary care and family practice front-line. Collectively, we covered from tower to trench.

After 30-plus years of combined experience working with obese patients, we have set out to write the book we each wish we'd had when we started out. Our goal was to create not a dry textbook with an overwhelming degree of minutia, but rather an immediately useful overview of the practical aspects of clinical obesity care, from the approach to the design of the physical office space to actual patient- and practice-based advice.

For some, this book may serve as a springboard for the establishment of an evidence-based weight-management practice, while for others it may simply allow them to feel more comfortable in their approach to treating obese patients. Most importantly, we hope that this book will stimulate health care professionals to remember that this is reality, not reality television — the concept of 'Best Weight' has far more value than any specific "ideal" or unrealistic body mass index (BMI).

With obesity serving as the last socially acceptable target of stereotypic scorn and discrimination, perhaps Dr. Mickey Stunkard said it best:

> "Here is a golden opportunity. As with any chronic illness, we rarely have the opportunity to cure. But we do have the opportunity to treat the patient with respect. Such an experience may be the greatest gift that a doctor can give an obese patient; it compares favorably with the modest benefits of our programs of weight reduction" (p. 356) Stunkard 1993; *Obesity: Theory and Therapy*]

Don't let that opportunity pass you by.

Sincerely,
Dr. Yoni Freedhoff, MD
Dr. Arya M. Sharma, MD, PhD

[CONTENTS]

[CHAPTER 1: OFFICE SET-UP]

Before we get into the whys and wherefores of weight management, let us briefly examine the environment in which you will be working.

THE WAITING ROOM

Your waiting room is the first thing patients see when they walk into your office, and it helps set the tone for your consultations. Trust and confidence are important aspects of the doctor-patient relationship, and a patient who feels you have considered their needs in the design of your waiting room may feel more comfortable initiating or responding to a discussion about weight control.

There are three main weight-related issues to consider when designing a waiting room: seating, available reading materials, and privacy.

Seating

Put simply, seating matters. Rows of narrow seats with armrests that risk trapping patients can be demoralizing. For your heavier patients' consideration, provide at least one bank of wide-based seats without armrests. While 24-inch-wide armless seats will suffice in most cases, it may be worthwhile to provide one or two specialized bariatric armchairs with double-width seats and sturdy armrests that serve as push-off points for patients who need the help of their arms to stand up.

Reading Materials

Your waiting room is filled with patients leafing through magazines. But what are they reading about? Obesity is a very hot topic in the media, and many publications feature articles about new miracle diets and weight-loss products and supplements. Patients may assume that you tacitly endorse these approaches to weight management — after all, they are reading about these products in your office. Clinic staff should regularly remove magazines that encourage unhealthy eating or fad diets or promote impossibly thin body ideals. It is best to stick with general interest magazines devoted to subjects like news, travel or nature, along with quality health publications.

Privacy

For most patients, weight is a very private matter. For some, it is a lifelong nemesis and unending source of anxiety. Make sure your office scale is tucked away in a low- or no-traffic area that offers at least a modicum of privacy. Check that it is not visible from the waiting room, or situated within earshot of staff and other patients. If staff members typically weigh your patients, instruct them to always ask the patient's permission first. A question such as, "Would it be all right if I weighed you?" instantly conveys the tone you want to establish — that you and your office understand and respect patients' sensitivities and needs, and will do your utmost to accommodate them. Doing so will set the tone for a thoughtful and compassionate interaction.

THE EXAMINING ROOM

Your examining room must contain equipment adapted to larger patients. A number of items require special consideration:

Gowns: Make sure you stock gowns suitable for bariatric patients. An examination in an ill-fitting, revealing gown is an endurance test for anyone, and modesty is especially important for patients struggling with body image. Accommodating larger patients with gowns that fit is a simple step that removes a potential stressor and facilitates the establishment of an empathetic rapport. Larger gowns have become easier to find; if your regular medical supply service does not have them available, ask your representative to track some down.

Scales: You need a scale capable of measuring weights of at least 226.8 kilograms (kg) or 500 pounds (lb). While expensive, a scale of this size is necessary if you are to treat the heaviest patients, who have the highest risk of serious attendant health problems. The message that your office is not even equipped to weigh them will seriously undermine your interactions. The scale should have a wide, supportive base and a readout mounted to one side so that both you and your patient have an unobstructed view.

> ▶ **Pearl:** Shipping scales are a reasonably priced alternative to medical-grade scales and are accurate enough for clinical purposes.

Blood pressure cuffs: While large-sized cuffs will serve most of your patient population, a small investment in a thigh-sized cuff will enable you take the blood pressure of even your heaviest patients. Using cuffs that are too small can lead to over-estimations of blood pressure, unnecessary prescriptions or increases in anti-hypertensive medications.

> ▶ **Pearl:** Reliable when properly used, newer blood pressure instruments designed for the wrist fit large patients better than arm cuffs and do not require the sometimes awkward exposing of the upper arm.

Examining tables: Ensure you have at least one extra-wide table large and strong enough for your heaviest patients. Provide an accompanying oversized step stool to help patients climb up, and place the table at least a few inches away from the wall so patients do not feel wedged in.

> ▶ **Pearl:** An examining table that is lower than usual (desk height or below) is easy for patients to get onto and provides a better vantage point for the exam.

GENERAL CONSIDERATIONS

Hallways: If you have the opportunity to design your office space, think about widening its passages so that bariatric patients do not feel they have to hug the wall to let someone by.

> ▶ **Pearl:** Bariatric wheelchairs, walkers and scooters require a door-width of at least 91.5 cm (36 inches) — wider than the average doorway (75 cm or 30 inches).

Bathrooms: You likely already have "grab bars" installed in handicapped-accessible bathrooms, but you may want to equip all of your office toilets with them. Standard toilets sit low to the floor and some bariatric patients may require grab bars to get back up. Consider installing toilets on raised platforms to make rising easier.

> ▶ **Pearl:** There is nothing worse than having a toilet break off the wall — try for a floor-mounted toilet, or install a toilet jack to add vertical support to your toilet's wall mount and increase its weight-bearing capacity.

[CHAPTER 2: LET'S TALK ABOUT WEIGHT]

While there are many ways to begin helping patients manage their weight, some work better than others. Many patients will not bring up the subject of weight loss on their own and may dread the idea of their doctor broaching the topic. In these circumstances, setting the right tone is an essential first step.

This chapter looks at good and bad ways to approach the subject of weight management. It begins with three common approaches we cannot recommend, then explores a more open-ended, collaborative approach designed to establish a rapport and earn your patient's trust.

WRONG APPROACH #1: SCARE TACTICS

"If you don't lose weight soon, you're going to kill yourself!"

Your patients know their weight puts them at risk — they experience its health impacts every day, which is why they are currently sitting in your office. Scaring a patient will only increase the insecurities they arrived with, and will do nothing to positively motivate them to change their situation. Willpower diminishes with a sense of failure, and even the most committed patient may initially balk at a weight-loss program because of feelings of inadequacy — after all, a lack of success in this area is what drove your patients to seek you out in the first place. Self-confidence is key, and scare tactics are never reassuring and may even paralyze patients into inaction. Given the drastic effort needed to lose weight, paralysis is the last thing you want to induce.

WRONG APPROACH #2: SLOGANS AND STOCK PHRASES

"Eat less; exercise more."

Slogans may work in mass advertising; they come off as trite with an audience of one. Nobody likes being patronized, which is the only thing these stock phrases achieve. Utter them and your patients will know for sure that you have absolutely no understanding of the complexities of their situation. If it were that easy, all your patients would be skinny, and we would not be writing this book.

WRONG APPROACH #3: GUILT

"Don't you care about your health?"

Backing your patient into the "guilt corner" only serves to erode the doctor-patient relationship. Guilt is something the severely obese already have in abundance.

A COLLABORATIVE APPROACH

"I'm sure you're aware that your weight can affect your health. Do you have any concerns about your weight and health that you'd like to talk about?"

Here, the approach is collaborative. You open the door to conversation, but allow your patient to steer where it will go. While a large percentage of patients with excess weight want to lose it, not all are ready to actually start making changes. The question above allows you to determine what stage of change your patient has reached. For the patient who has reached a pre-contemplation stage (see the section on page 10 on Readiness for Change), this open-ended approach might steer them towards contemplation. Those already contemplating a weight-loss effort may move to the next stage of preparation.

Table 1: What's in a name?

What words should you use to discuss your patient's weight? We know it is inappropriate to use the term *fat* to discuss weight with a patient, but is the term *obese* any better? Your patient's definition of obesity is likely quite different than your "BMI of 30 or more." When a patient hears the term *obese*, the image they conjure is one that would meet the definition of extreme morbid obesity, i.e., a BMI > 50.

Tom Wadden and Elizabeth Didie from the University of Pennsylvania and Drexel University studied the issue to find out "What's in a name? Patients' Preferred Terms for Describing Obesity." Their simple yet elegant study, published in *Obesity Research*, polled 167 obese women to rate 11 terms used to describe obesity on a scale from very undesirable to very desirable.

Obese Women (N = 167)

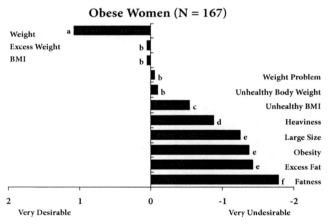

Source: **Wadden T., Didie, E.** What's in a Name? Patients' Preferred Terms for Describing Obesity. *Obesity Research* 11; 1140-1146: 2003.

Least desirable was the term *fatness*, followed closely by *excess fat* and *obesity*. The only term that rated favourably was the word *weight*.

On the other hand, the medical name for the disease is *obesity*, so do not shy away from the use of this term in your medical records or when communicating with colleagues.

Whether patients express interest in weight management after you initiate the discussion or start the discussion themselves, your first reaction should be to offer encouragement while gently probing their motives and goals. This is a good opportunity to determine whether your patient has realistic expectations and a plan for achieving their goals.

Ask "Why?" after patients state a desire to lose weight and they will certainly be surprised, but in a constructive way. More often than not they will explain their reasons or come back with a question such as "Don't you think I should?" This type of conversation provides a valuable opportunity to learn about your patient's motives and objectives.

Motivation: Aesthetics vs. Health

Aesthetics are a prime motivator for many people who want to lose weight. Do not make the mistake of equating this with superficiality before you have explored your patients' motivation a little further. While going to a wedding or fitting into a bathing suit may not seem a strong foundation for long-term resolve, aesthetic considerations such as increasing self-esteem, improving sex life, dressing better or finding a partner, are all strong and reasonable reasons for initiating weight-management efforts.

However, it is important to emphasize that while weight loss may help them achieve appearance-related goals, it is not a remedy for relationship difficulties or psychological issues. A patient motivated primarily by the desire to improve a relationship or increase self-esteem may be less likely to achieve weight-management goals than one motivated by health reasons.

> ▸ **Pearl:** If weight loss is driven mainly by concerns over body image and self-esteem, then these issues need to be addressed. It may help to point out to these patients that "weight cycling" is a sure-fire way to keep gaining weight.

If patients report improving health as their primary objective, we try to elicit specific examples of what should improve, such as increased energy or less knee pain. We then try to define objective quality-of-life or health goals that can be achieved within a reasonable time span; for one it may be to walk around the block or go to the mall, while for another it may be to reduce the need for blood pressure or pain medication. Sometimes short-term weight-loss goals for medical reasons can be reasonable objectives (e.g., weight loss prior to knee surgery). In all cases, success should be measured by the achievement of these goals rather than by the amount of weight actually lost. In fact, some of these goals, such as walking around the block or climbing stairs, can be achieved with no weight loss at all, just by increasing fitness. These successes should be highlighted.

> ▸ **Pearl:** The goal of weight loss should not be just to reduce numbers on a scale, but to reduce health risks and improve quality of life.

Motivation: Intrinsic vs. Extrinsic

Try to find out whether the motivation for weight loss comes from the patient themself or from someone else. If the desire is extrinsic, it is worth exploring why the patient feels that other person wants them to lose weight. Obesity treatment is unlikely to be successful unless the patient wants it themselves; losing weight to please someone else may not provide sufficient motivation, and may in fact cultivate eating-based oppositional defiance.

If the primary motivation is coming from within, it is important to know what kind of support system the patient can count on. Will their efforts be supported or sabotaged at home? How committed are partners to supporting the treatment effort? Is the family ready to change? Statements such as "We always have soda and chips in the house for the kids," "My mother-in-law always brings us food," or "My husband demands three cooked meals a day," can indicate a less-than-supportive environment. Friends can also play an important role. If a patient's circle of friends regularly centres social gatherings on eating, this will certainly have an impact on your patient's likelihood of success.

> ▸ **Pearl:** Patients should understand that while weight loss often results in positive medical and aesthetic outcomes, those outcomes are anything but guaranteed. We will often inform our patients that "The only guaranteed change if you lose weight is that you'll need smaller clothing — everything else is a bonus." Allowing a patient to entertain an unrealistic expectation is a recipe for disappointment.

Why Lose Weight Now?

It is worthwhile to try and understand a patient's timing. Is now really the best time? Weight loss requires considerable mental and physical effort. It may not be best to embark on a weight-management effort if the patient expects to be facing periods of stress or immobility in the near future. On the other hand, changes in circumstance, such as a new job or relationship, may provide a good opportunity to alter established patterns and habits that have perpetuated weight gain.

Readiness for Change

Prochaska's Readiness for Change model provides a reasonable guide for the clinician's efforts to advise patients about weight management. While there is little point in trying to convince someone who is at a pre-contemplation stage, carefully-worded advice to those in the preparation, action, maintenance and relapse stages can be highly effective. The patient who desires to lose weight has clearly reached at least the preparation stage, and may already be at the action stage. Understanding which stage of change a patient has reached is crucial for delivering advice and encouragement that can prompt, or sustain, a patient's efforts (see Table 2 on page 11).

Table 2: Prochaska's Readiness for Change model	
Pre-contemplation	Patient has no intention of changing behaviour in the foreseeable future (within next six months).
Contemplation	Patient is aware that a problem exists and is seriously thinking about overcoming it (within next six months).
Preparation	Patient is intending to take action in the next month. This phase combines intention and small behavioural changes.
Action	Patient modifies behaviour, experiences or environment to overcome the problem. It involves the most overt behavioural changes.
Maintenance	Patient works to prevent relapse and consolidate the gains attained during action.

Source: **Prochaska, J. O. et al.** In Search of How People Change: Applications to Addictive Behaviors. *American Psychologist* 47(9); 1102-1114: 1992.

GOALS

One of the first questions a patient will ask you as they embark on an intentional weight-loss effort is, "How much do you think I should weigh?" Unfortunately, there is no correct answer.

Patients often want to know their *ideal* weight or ideal BMI. While a variety of different classification schemes for obesity are available, their utility lies primarily in statistical analysis and research, not in the individual clinical encounter.

Telling a patient whose BMI is 50 that they need to lose virtually 50% of their present body weight to be healthy is an exceptionally unhelpful means of discussing weight. The patient may not have weighed that little in decades, and you will have only provided them with a goal that seems daunting if not wholly unattainable.

Waist circumference and waist-to-hip ratios are useful in ascertaining the medical risk a patient's weight presents, but are no better than BMI in terms of goal-setting.

Even a 5% weight loss has been shown to produce medically measurable results, so any amount of weight loss is helpful. In some cases, rapid weight loss over the first few weeks of a weight-management program, as induced by a very low-calorie* diet, can increase motivation. However, this rapid rate of weight loss cannot be maintained and is likely to lead to frustration later in the program. As with any obesity treatment, the maintenance of lean body mass is crucial and rapid weight loss has been shown to disproportionately affect lean tissue. If a patient insists on rapid weight loss, you may need to reassess their underlying motivations and expectations.

---

* *The term calorie(s) is used in place of kilocalorie(s) throughout the book , except in reference to specific quantities.*

> ▸ **Pearl:** Sustainability is far more important than the speed of weight loss, which is why we often tell patients it would be better for them to lose half as much weight and take four times longer to do so, than to lose it all quickly and regain every last gram and sometimes even more.

Best Weight

"Best weight" is a non-statistical goal that is easy to set and easy to explain to patients. Patients can diet themselves down to any weight they put their minds to, but to maintain that weight, they need to actually enjoy the lifestyle that got them there.

A patient's best weight is therefore whatever weight they achieve while living the healthiest lifestyle they can truly enjoy. There comes a point when a person cannot eat less or exercise more and still like their life. The weight they attain while still liking their life is thus their "best" weight, as without the addition of pharmacotherapy or a surgical intervention, no further weight loss will be possible.

We need to remember that in modern society, eating is not simply about survival. We use food for comfort and for celebration and, with the exception of religious prohibitions, there should be no forbidden foods. If your patient cannot use food to comfort or celebrate, or if they consider certain foods "forbidden," then they are likely on a diet, and unfortunately diets are known to fail over 95% of the time. For sustainable weight management, a patient should be consuming the smallest number of calories that still allows them to enjoy each day. Some days will simply warrant more calories, such as birthdays, anniversaries, religious holidays, and days when injuries, illness or fights with loved ones occur. Simply put, ice-cream and cookies and their cultural and ethnic equivalents are vital parts of a rich life experience.

With exercise, a patient should be encouraged to be as physically active as possible and include as much additional exercise as they can enjoy each day. Some days obviously will allow for more activity than others, but there is a maximum, above which the patient would run out of time or energy, hurt themselves or come to hate exercise. That is when they quit.

Eating less and exercising more within the context of a life the patient does not enjoy is the very definition of a diet, which is why diets almost always fail over the long-term. If a patient does not enjoy the way they are living while they are losing weight, they will almost certainly revert to "normal" practices and gain the weight back.

> ▸ **Pearl:** The difference between dieting and a healthy lifestyle is easy to explain. A diet is the smallest number of calories and the greatest amount of exercise that a patient can tolerate. A healthy lifestyle is the smallest number of calories and the greatest amount of exercise that a patient can enjoy.

Realistic vs. Unrealistic Expectations

Take a minute to conduct a reality check before your patient leaves the office. A realistic goal might be to achieve a 5%–10% weight loss at the rate of 0.5–1 kg (1–2 lbs) per week. It is important to emphasize the significant health benefits that can result from a 5%–10% weight loss. Unrealistic goals (e.g., 18 kg or 40 lbs in four weeks) reflect a lack of understanding of the basic principles of energy balance. As the patient's body becomes smaller, it also burns fewer calories. The initially large caloric deficit produces gradual weight loss but finally reaches a floor, whereupon the body settles into a new caloric equilibrium. Once patients reach this floor, they will need to find new ways to establish a caloric deficit if they want to lose more weight. A simple tool that plots the anticipated rate of weight loss and illustrates when they are likely to reach the floor is an effective management tool.

> ▸ **Pearl:** Your patients may talk about reaching a "plateau," but what they are most likely experiencing is a new caloric equilibrium: the floor. Patients may experience real plateaus during a weight management effort, where for weeks they see no further weight loss despite doing the same thing, but this generally reflects either an underestimation of caloric consumption, or that the scale is measuring something other than true weight, such as constipation, water retention or clothing. The laws of conservation of energy apply to people, and so long as your patients are eating fewer calories than they are burning, they must be losing weight.

HOW WILL YOU LOSE WEIGHT?

How does your patient plan to achieve weight loss? Most patients have some idea how they would like to achieve their goal. Some will have a positive plan, while others have thought more about what they are not willing to do, such as liquid diets, going to the gym or giving up soft drinks. Listen carefully to the patient's intentions, as these will help provide proper guidance.

Plan vs. No Plan?

The more specific a patient's plan, the greater the likelihood of success. A patient may state a plan to cut out soft drinks, snacks, or high-glycemic index (GI) foods. Patients with unrealistic plans involving approaches such as a cabbage-soup diet, a 10-day fast, or eating no food after 5 p.m., should be counselled on more appropriate strategies. The impact of what you say may be minimal, but it is better to try and discourage patients than do nothing. Patients who have no specific plan will need positive guidance. The question "What can you see yourself doing?" may be helpful.

Past Successes and Failures

Traditionally, the weight-loss component of obesity treatment has been relatively simple: all a patient had to do was suffer. Of course, if weight is lost through suffering, it will almost certainly be regained when your patient has decided that they have suffered enough and they revert to their original lifestyle.

Patients will often define success only in terms of the amount of weight lost. A more meaningful definition would be whether or not the weight loss was maintained.

We often advise patients to use the same approach that has worked for them in the past. However, it is important to explore why the patient abandoned that last effort. If a patient says, "It worked, but I hated it," new approaches should be discussed. The vast majority of your patients will regain some, if not all, of the weight they lose. While a large part of this is likely due to a patient's inability to sustain lifelong lifestyle changes, it is also partly due to the fact that our biology is designed to protect our weight and ensure that any lost weight is regained.

This is a good time to discuss the need for ongoing treatment once weight loss is achieved. To emphasize this point, we sometimes tell patients, "Maybe you should go and lose some weight and then come back for obesity treatment." They should understand that the more weight they would like to permanently lose, the more of their lifestyles they will need to permanently change. And lifestyle changes alone may be insufficient — some patients will require the ongoing use of partial meal replacements and/or medication as adjunctive treatments. As with any other chronic medical condition, the cessation of treatment will result in the recurrence of the condition. If a patient ceases any aspect of their obesity treatment (lifestyle changes and/or partial meal replacements and/or medications), their excess weight will likely recur.

In some cases the only successful treatment may be surgical, but even surgical weight management approaches require sustained lifestyle changes and, sometimes, medications.

Unfortunately, there is currently no "cure" for obesity: whatever treatment is chosen, it will have to be continued forever — treatments that are not sustainable do not result in sustainable weight loss.

▸ **Pearl:** Tell your patients,

"If you do not like the way you are living while you are losing your weight, you will almost certainly re-gain the weight when you go back to the way you were living before you lost it."

This simple statement may help steer them away from unsafe, non-sustainable and sometimes extremely expensive commercial programs and fad diets.

[CHAPTER 3: TREATMENT HURDLES]

Before recommending weight management programs or strategies, it is important to identify and deal with barriers that may make weight loss more difficult for particular patients, or undermine their efforts at weight-loss maintenance. Pre-emptive management of these barriers can increase the likelihood of long-term success and protect the patient from the emotional and physical consequences of weight cycling.

HURDLE 1: OBESITY IS NOT RECOGNIZED AS A CHRONIC CONDITION

Even among health care professionals, there is a pervasive attitude that obesity is simply a failure of individual willpower rather than a condition that requires chronic treatment. As a result, patients too often fail to accept the need for long-term lifestyle changes, medication and/or surgery, and health care professionals too often fail to recommend them.

Educating both patients and health care workers is essential to increase awareness of the chronicity of obesity as a disease, thereby improving adherence and increasing the recommendation of long-term treatments.

Many people believe that there is in fact a cure for obesity: simply lose the weight. They forget that the more difficult component of weight management is actually keeping the weight off. Patients are usually prepared to go through the first stage and reduce their weight, but they are not prepared to assume the life-long measures needed to maintain that weight loss.

HURDLE 2: SOCIO-ECONOMIC STATUS

Socio-economic factors are closely associated with obesity. This relationship is complex: just as socio-economic status may influence obesity, obesity may influence socio-economic status, and common factors may influence both. In developing countries, obesity is associated with higher socio-economic status, while in developed countries, low income and low education have been associated with both obesity and weight-related co-morbidities.

Changes in diet and activity levels may be more difficult to accomplish for people of lower socio-economic status. Lower income makes it difficult to afford healthy foods (i.e., lean meat cuts, fruits and vegetables can be more expensive than cereals and foods that are rich in fat and sugar). As well, medications and surgical interventions for obesity may not be covered by public health plans.

Individuals from lower-income strata may not be able to afford access to exercise facilities or organized sports programs, and may lack time for discretionary physical activity. Other barriers to exercise can include a lack of social support, the physical limitations of excess weight, a dislike for or medical inability to participate in vigorous exercise, embarrassment and past unpleasant experiences. Some may find it easier to incorporate more physical activity into to their daily lives (e.g., using stairs instead of elevators, walking to work or parking a couple of blocks from work, etc.) than to commit to scheduled exercise sessions.

HURDLE 3: TIME

Lack of time is one of the most common barriers to persisting with a weight management strategy. Planning a healthy diet, preparing home-cooked meals and exercising all require a significant investment of time. It bears repeating: patients need to recognize that obesity is a chronic disease that has no "cure," that long-term treatment is necessary, and that this treatment involves permanent changes to their daily routines.

The weight management strategy you design with a patient must therefore be simple, enjoyable and adapted to their particular schedule so they can follow it over the long-term.

The time required will vary from one patient to the next, but it is safe to assume that a patient who is unable to commit to 30 minutes per day of combined dietary and fitness effort will be unlikely to succeed with weight management using a purely behavioural strategy. Asking patients whether they feel they can find 30 minutes a day for their weight management effort will help to assess their readiness and willingness to change.

Patients looking for quick fixes from pharmacological or surgical assistance must be reminded that dietary changes and physical activity are just as essential with pharmacological and surgical treatment as they are without them. Pharmacological treatment without lifestyle changes produces only very modest weight loss: 1.8 to 2.7 kgs (4 to 6 lbs) on average. Patients who undergo surgery have to be able to devote a significant amount of their time to shopping for, preparing and eating appropriate meals. If they cannot find the time to do this, they will be unable to achieve and maintain good results with either medication or surgery.

HURDLE 4: SABOTEURS

Weight-management efforts can be sabotaged in many ways. Support from partners, family and peers is often essential to coping with the long-term lifestyle changes needed for sustained weight maintenance. Unfortunately, close friends and family too often undermine a patient's weight-loss efforts. The sabotage may be unintentional, as with a group of friends whose only means of socializing is to meet for dinner in a particular restaurant. Other times, friends or family may feel threatened by the patient's decision to lose weight and the effect they expect this decision to have on their own lives. A jealous spouse, for example, may be concerned that a partner is attempting to lose weight to attract a new mate, or that he or she will attract more competing attention after losing weight.

If a patient's spouse appears to be posing a barrier to weight management, it may be worth inviting them into the office to discuss their concerns. An open discussion may help reduce resistance.

Well-intentioned spouses on the other hand can act like "food police," looking over their mate's shoulder at meals and asking whether or not they are "allowed to eat that." These spouses need to understand that the only question they ought to ask their partner is: "Is there any way I can help you?" Intrusive questions risk triggering oppositional defiance. Exploring your patient's perceptions of how friends and family may undermine their efforts at the outset of a weight management program may enable you to help reduce any negative effects.

Social and professional obligations can also sabotage a patient's efforts, as participation in activities centred on food and alcohol may be important for both personal and professional success. Someone whose job involves "wining and dining" potential clients may find sustainable weight loss very difficult.

Support, counselling and motivation from the medical team are essential, particularly during the weight maintenance period when the initial motivation to lose weight has decreased and the patient receives less positive reinforcement from watching the needle go down on the scale and hearing positive comments from friends and family.

HURDLE 5: IATROGENIC CONTRIBUTIONS

Any number of medications can promote weight gain or hinder weight loss. A thorough medication review can lead to beneficial changes in medications; the exercise itself can enhance the doctor-patient relationship, as it demonstrates a desire to help. However, weight-neutral alternatives are not often available. When prescribing adipogenic medications, take the time to counsel patients regarding the possibility of iatrogenic weight gain, and discuss measures they might employ to prevent it. The following list is by no means comprehensive, but it does include the culprits most commonly seen in general practice.

Hypoglycemics

Improved glycemic control achieved through the administration of insulin, insulin secretagogues or thiazolidinediones (TZDs) is generally accompanied by weight gain. Weight gain on insulin secretagogues and insulin has been associated with increased blood pressure and lipids.

> ▸ **Pearl:** The weight gain associated with TZDs generally results from subcutaneous fat build-up. TZDs also cause a redistribution of fat from visceral to subcutaneous depots, which leads to improvements in metabolic parameters.

Antipsychotics

Weight gain is a well-documented side effect of antipsychotic treatment. It is generally not proportional to dose, and can vary from 1 kg–5 kg (2.2 lbs–11 lbs) over several years to enormous gains over just a few months. Both typical and novel antipsychotics are associated with weight gain, but novel antipsychotics, especially clozapine and olanzapine, have the greatest adipogenic potential and carry the greatest risk for the development of hypertension, diabetes and lipid abnormalities.

Table 3: Average weight gain with selected novel antipsychotics	
Atypical Antipsychotic	Average weight gain
Olanzapine	2–3 kg (4.5–6.5 lbs) per month
Clozapine	1.7 kg (3.7 lbs) per month
Quetiapine	1.8 kg (4 lbs) per month
Risperidone	1 kg (2.2 lbs) per month

Source: **Wetterling, T.** Body weight gain with atypical antipsychotics. A comparative review. *Drug Safety* 24; 59-73: 2001.

Of all the novel antipsychotics, ziprasidone and aripiprazole appear to be nearly weight neutral.

While we would not recommend discontinuing antipsychotic medications in patients who suffer from psychosis, these medications are increasingly used off-label as mood stabilizers and sleep aids. If your patient does not require an antipsychotic for the treatment of psychosis, consider stopping treatment and exploring less obesogenic alternatives.

> ▸ **Pearl:** A recent study suggests that the co-administration of metformin with antipsychotic medications may attenuate iatrogenic weight gain. Metformin's effect was heightened when combined with behavioural weight-management strategies.

Antidepressants

Tricyclic antidepressants are often associated with weight gain. Amitriptyline appears to have the greatest obesogenic potential. Reduced energy expenditure appears to be behind the weight-promoting effect of these drugs, while changes in food intake contribute to a smaller extent. Selective serotonin reuptake inhibitors (SSRIs) are not generally obesogenic, but in rare cases they can produce significant weight gain.

> ▸ **Pearl:** The weight gain associated with antidepressants cannot be explained solely by improvement in depressive symptoms.

Weight gain is also common with lithium treatment; it appears to be dose-related, and is more likely to occur in women who are already overweight.

Anticonvulsants

Weight gain is one of the most common effects of antiepileptic drugs, in particular valproate and carbamazepine. These drugs are used in the treatment of both epilepsy and bipolar disorder. In susceptible individuals, the weight gain, which is generally tied to increased food intake, can be so pronounced as to require discontinuation of the medication.

> ▸ **Pearl:** Lamotrigine is a weight-neutral antiepileptic drug, while topiramate and zonisamide may induce weight loss.

Steroids

Weight gain is a common adverse effect of long-term treatment with glucocorticoids. These drugs also increase abdominal adiposity: an effect that, combined with the increased insulin resistance steroids produce, may serve to explain the clear relationship between long-term glucocorticoid use and heightened risk for diabetes and cardiovascular disease.

Beta-Blockers

Treatment with non-selective beta-blockers has been associated with modest but sustained weight gain. The effect is thought to be mediated by a reduction in energy expenditure. It may be prudent to avoid beta-blockers in patients who do not have absolute indications (e.g., post myocardial infarction, congestive heart failure, tachyarrhythmias, etc.) for these drugs.

Highly Active Anti-Retroviral Therapy (HAART)

Although generally associated with weight loss, HAART can promote a redistribution of body fat from subcutaneous to visceral depots. Metabolic syndrome associated with abdominal adiposity is thus a common complication of anti-retroviral treatment. The accumulation of abdominal fat can lead to non-compliance with anti-retroviral medications in some patients.

HURDLE 6: SUBSTANCE ABUSE

Tobacco

Many patients are hesitant to try to quit smoking and undertake a weight-management effort simultaneously. Indeed, smoking cessation is associated with small amounts of weight gain, but the benefits of smoking cessation clearly outweigh the risk of gaining a few pounds.

If a patient is interested in quitting smoking but is also concerned about weight gain, buproprion may be a reasonable pharmacologic aid. Buproprion is associated with weight loss when used in the treatment of depression and may blunt the weight gain associated with smoking cessation.

Alcohol

Alcohol is a significant source of calories. At 7 kcal per gram, one large glass of wine a night adds up to 65,700 kcal per year (the equivalent of nearly 9 kg [20 lbs] in weight gain), and has no effect on satiety. In most situations, there is no compensatory reduction in other calories consumed. Alcohol can produce a positive fat balance, as it has a sparing effect on fat oxidation and promotes fat storage. Alcohol is also an appetite stimulant, often used as an aperitif, and has a tendency to reduce a person's resolve. Many patients consider their glass of wine to be a heart-healthy habit, but if they are not at a healthy weight, the health risk of additional calories outweighs the potential benefits of moderate drinking.

Marijuana and Hashish

Cannabis users may experience weight gain due to increased appetite ("the munchies") and caloric intake, as the drug stimulates cannabinoid receptor–1 (CN1) activity. These receptors are found in several areas of the brain, including the hypothalamus, where appetite and satiety are regulated. Because of this effect on appetite, long-term weight management may prove far more difficult for regular cannabis users.

Blocking the CN1 receptor has been proposed as a novel mechanism to reduce appetite and treat obesity. A number of drug companies pursued CN1 receptor antagonists in clinical weight management, however, due to an unexpectedly high rate of psychiatric side effects they have been withdrawn from use worldwide.

Illicit Drugs

Obesity has not been specifically associated with an increased risk of illicit drug abuse. However, it is important to identify and treat dependencies on illicit drugs before starting a weight-management plan.

Diuretics and Laxatives

The use of diuretics and laxatives should be investigated. These drugs are frequently used for purging by patients with eating disorders, which should always be treated before starting a weight-management plan.

HURDLE 7: SYNDROMAL OBESITY

Syndromal forms of obesity pose an important challenge to treatment. A large number of syndromes are associated with childhood-onset obesity. These include obesity as a clinical feature and are often associated with mental retardation, dysmorphic features and organ-specific developmental abnormalities. While there is some evidence to support the use of meal replacements, very low-calorie diets, medications and even surgery in these patients, no long-term efficacy studies have been conducted to date.

Prader-Willi Syndrome

Prader-Willi syndrome is the most common syndromal cause of obesity, with an estimated prevalence of about 1 in 25,000. It is an autosomal dominant disorder characterized by diminished fetal activity, obesity, hypotonia, mental retardation, short stature, hypo-gonadotropic hypogonadism, and small hands and feet. Hyperphagia is a dominant feature in Prader-Willi syndrome.

Bardet-Biedl Syndrome

Bardet-Biedl syndrome is a rare autosomal recessive disease characterized by obesity, mental retardation, dysmorphic extremities (syndactyly, brachydactyly or polydactyly), retinal dystrophy or pigmented retinopathy, hypogonadism or hypogenitalism (limited to male patients) and structural abnormalities of the kidney or functional renal impairment.

Other Genetic Disorders

Albright's hereditary osteodystrophy is an autosomal dominant disorder characterized by short stature, obesity, skeletal defects, and impaired olfaction.

More recently, several human single-gene disorders, such as leptin deficiency, pro-opiomelanocortin (POMC) deficiency and melanocortin-4 receptor (MC4R) deficiency, have been identified. These mutations all result in morbid obesity in childhood with-out the development of the pleiotropic features characteristic of recognized childhood obesity syndromes. The most common of these gene disorders is MC4R deficiency, which has no pathognomonic features. The diagnosis should be considered in cases of early onset familial obesity, usually with clear dominant inheritance.

[CHAPTER 4: PSYCHIATRIC BARRIERS]

It is helpful to remind patients that obesity most often results from normal behaviour in an abnormal environment. Psychopathologies are not more common in obese individuals than in non-obese individuals. Psychosocial issues and psychiatric disorders can, however, predispose individuals to obesity and/or create significant barriers to treatment. As well, many of the medications used to treat psychiatric disorders may iatrogenically contribute to weight gain or difficulty with weight loss. Underlying emotional and psychiatric disorders that can contribute to the development and persistence of obesity need to be addressed if a weight-management program is to be effective.

Many different psychiatric and emotional disorders can promote weight gain or obstruct weight loss. Treatment of these co-morbidities may be needed before initiating a weight-management strategy.

Failure to recognize these barriers to treatment will reduce the likelihood of success in weight management, which can in turn aggravate problems of low self-esteem, anxiety or depression, and perpetuate emotional and psychiatric problems.

Patients with suspected emotional or psychiatric disorders may require referral for further evaluation and treatment before embarking on a weight-management plan.

EATING DISORDERS

A wide range of abnormal eating behaviours, ranging from simply skipping meals (disordered eating) to full-blown DSM-diagnosable binge-eating disorders, can pose significant barriers to obesity treatment. While some of these disorders can be dealt with as part of the obesity-management strategy, severe eating disorders require specialized behavioural interventions that are generally beyond the scope of general practice. Such patients should be referred to an eating disorder specialist before you initiate a weight-management program.

Binge-Eating Disorder

Binge eating, also called compulsive overeating, is probably the most common eating disorder and is present in 2% of all adults. Among mildly obese people in self-help or commercial weight-loss programs, 10% to 15% have a binge-eating disorder, and prevalence rises to as much as 40% among those with severe obesity. Binge-eating disorder is slightly more common in women, with three women affected for every two men.

Obese people with binge-eating disorder often became overweight at a younger age than those without the disorder. They may also have more frequent episodes of losing and regaining weight (weight cycling).

> ▸ **Pearl:** Binge-eating disorder should be suspected and investigated in patients with a history of frequent, marked and rapid weight cycling.

Binge eating is different from normal increases in appetite and occasional or contextual overeating (e.g., holiday meals). This disorder is also different from binge-purge syndrome (bulimia nervosa) because people with binge-eating disorder do not usually purge afterward by vomiting or using laxatives. People with a binge-eating problem eat unusually large amounts of food and do not stop eating when they become full. They binge regularly and describe feeling out of control and powerless to stop eating. Binge episodes may be triggered by negative emotions such as stress, anxiety, hurt, frustration, anger, sadness or boredom. Many find it comforting and soothing to eat food at such times, but after a binge they are likely to feel guilty and sad about their lack of control. People with binge-eating disorder are extremely distressed by their binge eating and often have very low self-esteem. Many have a history of emotional, physical or sexual abuse or unresolved grief. They usually rate their social environment regarding relationships as less supportive and cohesive.

Some people miss work, school or social activities in order to binge eat. Obese people with binge-eating disorder often feel badly about themselves, are preoccupied with their appearance, and may avoid social gatherings. Most feel ashamed and try to hide their problem. They are often so successful that close family members and friends do not know about their binge eating. Most will have tried to control it on their own, but will have had only short-term success.

The causes of binge eating disorder are still unknown. Up to half of all people with binge-eating disorder have a history of depression, but whether depression is a cause or consequence of the disorder is unclear. Impulsive behaviour and certain other psychological problems may be more common in people with binge-eating disorder. The relationship between binge eating and childhood abuse, post-traumatic stress and unresolved grief is addressed below.

Although binge eating is strongly associated with a history of dieting, it is unclear whether dieting actually promotes binge-eating disorder. While findings vary, early research suggests that about half of all people with binge-eating disorder had binge episodes before they started dieting. However, strict dieting may worsen binge eating.

People who are not overweight or who are only mildly obese should avoid strict dieting, as it may worsen binge eating. However, many people with the disorder are severely obese and have medical problems related to their weight, making losing weight and keeping it off important treatment goals.

> ▸ **Pearl:** Ensure that patients with binge-eating disorder are not placed on a diet with less than 1400–1500 kcal per day, as more restrictive diets may exacerbate their binge eating.

Several studies have found that people with binge-eating disorder find it harder to comply with obesity treatment. Binge eaters are also more likely to regain weight quickly. For these reasons, people with the disorder may require treatment that focuses on their binge eating before they begin obesity treatment. Normal-weight patients who are frequently distressed by their binge eating may also benefit from treatment.

Several methods are currently used to treat binge-eating disorder. Cognitive-behavioural therapy teaches patients techniques to monitor and change their eating habits and how they cope with difficult situations. Interpersonal psychotherapy helps people examine their relationships with friends and family, and make changes when problems are identified. Treatment with medications such as antidepressants may be helpful for some individuals. Self-help groups can also be a source of support. The choice of treatment should be discussed with the patient and a mental health professional with experience in this area.

Table 4: Diagnosis of binge-eating disorder

Binge-eating episodes occur, on average, at least two days a week for six months and are associated with at least three of the following:

- Eating much more rapidly than normal
- Eating until feeling uncomfortably full
- Eating large amounts of food when not feeling physically hungry
- Eating alone due to embarrassment at how much one is eating
- Feeling disgusted with oneself, depressed, or very guilty after overeating
- Marked distress about the binge-eating behaviour

Source: **Tanosky-Kraff et al.** Eating disorder or disordered eating? Nonnormative eating patterns in obese individuals. *Obesity Research* 12;1361-1366: 2004.

Homeostatic or Hedonic Binging?

In our experience, the majority of patients who struggle with binge-eating episodes do not eat regularly throughout the day, and tend to struggle with binge behaviours from mid-afternoon onward. In these patients, the binge is likely precipitated by true physical or homeostatic hunger (a need for calories) rather than a hedonistic emotional need for comfort foods (appetite). Well-distributed calories and the use of more satiating protein-rich foods may be enough to resolve the disorder in these patients.

The difference between patients with homeostatic and hedonic binge-eating disorder is so marked that we wonder whether the presence of meal or snack-skipping should be included in the upcoming DSM-V (estimated release: May, 2012) as an exclusionary criterion for the diagnosis of binge-eating disorder.

Before diagnosing someone with binge-eating disorder, you should first ensure that a subtle form of homeostatic hunger is not triggering or encouraging their behaviour. Have patients follow the eating instructions below to see whether their binge eating resolves:

- Breakfast containing a minimum of 350 kcal with at least 15 g of protein, to be consumed within 30 minutes of waking
- Snacking every 2.5 hours between meals with snacks containing 100–200 kcal and at least 8 g of protein
- Lunch containing a minimum of 300–400 kcal with at least 15 g of protein
- Dinner containing a minimum of 400 kcal with at least 15 g of protein
- For every hour of sustained exercise, add an additional 100–150 kcal that are primarily carbohydrate based

Night-Eating Syndrome

Night eating is increasingly recognized as a syndrome with distinct psychopathology. The sleep disturbance and increased food intake later in the day associated with night eating may contribute to weight gain and poorer weight-loss outcomes. Night eating syndrome (NES) is not the equivalent of night snacking.

Diagnostic criteria include:
- Skipping breakfast ≥ 4 days/week, interpreted as morning anorexia
- Consuming more than 50% of total daily calories after 7 p.m.
- Difficulty falling asleep or staying asleep ≥ 4 days/week

NES patients report more nocturnal awakenings and consume food during approximately 75% of awakenings vs. 0% for people without NES. Night eaters report more depression, lower self-esteem, less hunger and also more fullness before a daytime test meal. While the total energy intake of people with NES may not be different from that of over-weight or obese individuals without the syndrome, they consume more than three times as many calories after the evening meal.

DEPRESSION

Several studies have suggested a link between obesity and depression, especially in women, though it is unclear which comes first. Severe obesity in adults is associated with a five-fold increased risk for major depression, though there have been some con-flicting reports. While increased body weight has been associated with major depression, suicide attempts, and suicidal ideation in women, a large Swedish study found a strong inverse association between BMI and suicide in men: for each 5 kg/m^2 increase in BMI, the risk of suicide decreased by 15%. In severely obese adolescents,clinically significant levels of depressive symptoms are uncommon, despite global and severe impairment of day-to-day life. On the other hand, children and adolescents with major depressive disorder may be at increased risk of becoming overweight.

Patients with mood disorders may present with a depressed or irritable mood and/or a lack of normal interest in daily life. Depression may also present with the full DSM-IV gamut of symptoms, including change in appetite and weight, motor agitation or retardation, feelings of worthlessness or guilt, decreased ability to make decisions or concentrate, and recurrent thoughts of death and suicide. Yet diagnosing depression may not be as straightforward in obese patients, who can exhibit symptoms as a result of their over-all situation rather than organic depression. Many of these patients believe that their mood disorder is a consequence of their obesity and turn to food for comfort.

It is important to address both depression and obesity in the treatment plan. The primary focus should be on managing the depression as depressive anhedonia which, coupled with decreased concentration, can have a significant impact on a patient's motivation and ability to change lifestyle and behaviour. Inadequately treated depression should probably be considered a relative contraindication to initiating a purely lifestyle-based weight-management effort, as both concentration and organization are required for new habit cultivation.

In certain cases, treating obesity can indeed alleviate depression. It is, however, rare for the treatment of depression to alleviate obesity, and pharmacological treatment of depression may iatrogenically contribute to weight gain. Patients undergoing pharmacologic antidepressant treatment must be counselled on the possibility of weight gain and prophylactic behavioural or medical treatment may be required to prevent the development or exacerbation of obesity. Compared with tricyclic antidepressants, selective serotonin reuptake inhibitors (SSRIs) have much less impact on weight and bupropion has been associated with weight loss. Consideration of obesity in the choice of antidepressant may therefore lead to better adherence to therapy.

ABUSE, NEGLECT AND POST-TRAUMATIC STRESS

Childhood maltreatment or adverse experiences in five domains (emotional abuse, physical abuse, sexual abuse, emotional neglect and physical neglect) have been reported as highly prevalent in patients with binge-eating syndrome. In one study, 83% of patients with binge eating reported some form of childhood maltreatment: 59% reported emotional abuse, 36% reported physical abuse, 30% reported sexual abuse, 69% reported emotional neglect, and 49% reported physical neglect.

Maltreatment, notably emotional abuse and neglect, is significantly associated with depression and low self-esteem, but its relationship to weight, the onset of obesity or to other obesity-related features is less straightforward. Weight may be used by patients (consciously or unconsciously) as a way to push away the world or intimacy.

Post-traumatic stress disorder occurs in a subgroup of individuals exposed to a severe life-threatening trauma. The core set of symptoms are: intrusive re-experiencing, avoidance and arousal. Co-morbid substance abuse and mood and anxiety disorders are common. Trauma-exposed individuals are more likely to engage in behaviours that present a health risk and are more likely to report physical symptoms and functional impairment. A high prevalence of overweight and obesity is found in patients with post-traumatic stress disorder.

It is important to monitor patients with a history of abuse for recurrence of emotions or memories as they lose weight. Before initiating a weight-loss strategy, the possibility of weight-loss distress should be discussed with the patient. This is not an uncommon occurrence and the patient should know you are willing to discuss it with them.

ATTENTION DEFICIT DISORDER

Attention deficit disorder with or without hyperactivity (ADD or ADHD) and impulsiveness has been associated with increased risk for weight gain in both children and adults. In one study, ADHD was present in over 25% of all obese patients and 40% of patients with class III obesity. Reasons for this prevalent co-morbidity are unknown, but brain dopamine or insulin receptor activity may be involved.

Patients with ADD or ADHD usually manifest a long history (since childhood) of impulsivity, lack of concentration, decreased attention, inability to complete tasks, impairment in school or work performance and social dysfunction. Being "hyperactive" in the sense of the DSM-IV diagnosis of ADHD does not prevent the development or persistence of overweight and obesity in children.

Bariatric patients showing poor focus during treatment should be investigated for ADD or ADHD. Identifying the disorder is crucial as they will not be able to focus on the weight-management plan until their impulsiveness and lack of concentration are addressed.

Pharmacological and behavioural therapies can often help patients improve task persistence and decrease impulsivity and distractibility, which will increase the likelihood of success with weight-control efforts.

SEASONAL AFFECTIVE DISORDER

Seasonal affective disorder (SAD) is a recurring depression with seasonal onset and remission. SAD primarily occurs in the winter months and it is postulated that the decrease in daylight hours alters circadian rhythms and affects melatonin and serotonin levels.

A number of factors distinguish SAD from major depressive disorder. Especially important here is that SAD is often associated with increased rather than decreased appetite.

There are two primary treatment modalities for SAD. Light therapy involves exposure to visible light that produces a minimum of 2,500 lux at eye level. Daily treatment duration depends on the intensity of the light: two hours a day are needed with a light emitting 2,500 lux, while 30 minutes a day is sufficient with 10,000 lux. Light therapy devices are readily available in specialty health-care stores and on the Internet. SAD can also be treated with pharmacotherapy using antidepressants in the same way one would treat non-seasonal depression.

To date, no study has demonstrated additional benefit from combining light therapy and pharmacotherapy.

STRESS

Stress has both a psychological and physiological impact on weight management as it affects a patient's eating and exercise behaviours.

Physiologically, stress increases serum cortisol, which in turn affects appetite. Eating can be an appropriate response to stress as it decreases serum cortisol levels.

Psychologically, stressed individuals may find themselves more distractible with decreased ability to focus, concentrate and plan — abilities that are essential to lifestyle-based weight management. As well, individuals under stress may fall into more disorganized patterns of eating and miss meals or snacks, thereby allowing hunger to influence their eating decisions.

Teaching patients stress-reduction techniques, or directing them to appropriate stress-reduction resources may help with their weight-management efforts. Meditation, yoga, deep-breathing techniques, exercise and professional counselling can all be considered.

PSYCHOSIS

Symptoms suggestive of mania or psychosis need to be investigated and treated before initiating a weight-reduction strategy. Unfortunately, current pharmacotherapy for bipolar disorder (lithium, valproate, olanzapine) and many of the the newer antipsychotics (clozapine, olanzapine, quetiapine) can produce dramatic weight gains. This effect on body weight can exacerbate obesity-related illnesses and hinder compliance with antipsychotic treatment.

There has been some success using topiramate for bipolar and mood disorders both as an independent weight-neutral or even weight-negative mood stabilizer, and as an adjunct to other antipsychotics to decrease iatrogenic weight gain. Lamotrigine may also be considered as a mood stabilizer, and it too has been shown to be weight neutral.

Of all the novel antipsychotics, ziprasidone and aripiprazole have been reported to be nearly weight neutral.

Table 5: Antipsychotics and potential for weight gain	
Drug	**Degree of potential weight gain**
Molindone, Ziprasidone	-
Fluphenazine, Haloperidol, Risperidone	+
Chlorpromazine, Sertindole, Thioridazine, Mesoridazine	++
Olanzapine, Clozapine	+++

Source: Adapted from Allison, David B. et al. Antipsychotic-Induced Weight Gain: A Comprehensive Research Synthesis. *American Journal of Psychiatry* 156, 11; 1686-1696: 1999.

PERSONALITY TRAITS

There is no evidence that obese individuals share a particular personality profile. The heterogeneity in personality traits is comparable to that found in the general population. Nevertheless, certain personality traits can constitute barriers to obesity management. These may need to be addressed through appropriate counselling before initiating a weight-management intervention.

BODY IMAGE

The term body image refers to the collective perceptions, beliefs, assumptions and feelings we possess about our body and physical appearance.

Many people seeking help with weight management suffer from poor body image, and this can sabotage medically significant weight management when patients feel they have failed. The sense of failure may well see patients abandon their efforts completely and puts them at risk of gaining back all the weight they have lost — and often even more.

Body image starts to form very early and is influenced by the home environment, schoolyard experiences, personal relationships and mass media. Studies have reported that half of girls aged six to 18 want to be thinner. Other studies have demonstrated that weight-related stigmatization can start as early as age three.

> ▸ **Pearl:** Sudden changes in a patient's perception of their body image should alert you to the possibility of sexual abuse.

Identifying patients in your practice with poor body image is important as body image dissatisfaction is one of the strongest predictors of disordered eating behaviours. Certainly, if you have children in your practice whose parents are preoccupied with their body size or shape, it would be prudent to screen for eating disorders in the children and steer their parents to resources that can help them cultivate healthy eating behaviours and body image. While a full discussion of body image is beyond the scope of this book, some treatment tips will be provided in the behavioural interventions section of Chapter 6. We will discuss body image further in Chapter 8.

[CHAPTER 5: MEDICAL BARRIERS]

Physical co-morbidities are common in people with obesity and need to be addressed as part of any weight-management plan. Co-morbidities associated with obesity will improve as weight is controlled, but often make it difficult for patients to undertake the effort required for lifestyle-based weight management. In some cases, these physical barriers to weight loss may be insurmountable and the focus of treatment should, from the outset, aim to prevent weight gain rather than achieve weight loss. Strategies for obesity treatment should always be adapted to the patient's particular situation to make it easier for them to cope with required changes over the long-term.

SLEEP DISORDERS

Sleep disorders are very prevalent among obese people. Obstructive sleep apnea is the most common disorder, but disturbed sleep may also be due to primary insomnia, or insomnia secondary to medications, medical or psychiatric disorders.

Sleep deprivation is linked to obesity. The primary putative connection can be found in the neuroendocrine regulation of appetite and food intake. Neuroendocrine regulation appears to be influenced by sleep duration and sleep restriction, with sleep deprivation favouring obesity as it increases serum cortisol and decreases serum leptin levels. Another reason for the sleep disorder-obesity connection may be simply that the more time a person spends awake, the more time they have in which to eat.

Insufficient sleep causes important neurocognitive changes such as excessive daytime sleepiness, fatigue and altered mood. These may, in turn, have a significant impact on the patient's ability to persist with healthy lifestyle changes such as increasing their level of physical activity or taking the time to cook a healthy meal.

CHRONIC PAIN CONDITIONS

Any condition that leads to chronic pain can contribute to obesity by increasing physiological and psychological stress. Pain also makes exercise more difficult to undertake and enjoy.

Osteoarthritis and Back Pain

Obesity is commonly associated with musculoskeletal pain and osteoarthritis, resulting in functional and motor limitations. Obese patients usually move more slowly, are less flexible and feel pain when performing tasks at floor level. There is a strong association between knee osteoarthritis and obesity. Degenerative arthritis resulting from chronic trauma associated with excess body weight develops primarily in weight-bearing joints such as the knee and ankle. However osteoarthritis can also be seen in non-weight-bearing joints, suggesting a systemic inflammatory response. Excess body weight is also closely related to lower back pain. Both static and compressive loading may damage the integrity of intervertebral discs. Increased biomechanical force can also cause muscle sprain and ligament strain.

The presence of significant pain can promote immobility, leading to loss of muscle mass and reduced cardiopulmonary fitness. This can precipitate psychological and metabolic changes that promote further weight gain.

Patients with painful joints may benefit from water-based (non-weight-bearing) exercise and may require pain management before embarking on a weight-loss program. Obese patients requiring joint-replacement surgery are generally advised to lose weight (often in unrealistic amounts) before surgery, but this is very difficult if they are already partially immobilized by pain.

To complicate matters further, most commercial gyms are ill-equipped to handle the needs of obese clients, many of whom cannot go from lying down on the floor to standing up without assistance. Step classes and aerobics classes are in many cases ill-advised, and exercise machines and weight benches are not usually designed for obese users.

Fibromyalgia
Obesity is often associated with fibromyalgia, a common disorder characterized by fatigue, pain, stiffness in the trunk and extremities and a number of specific tender points. Fibromyalgia is more common in women than in men and is frequently accompanied by sleep disorders. Treatment of fibromyalgia may increase a patient's ability to be physically active, and exercise has been shown to reduce the severity of fibromyalgia symptoms over time. As with severe osteoarthritis, starting with joint-sparing exercises may be prudent.

CARDIOVASCULAR AND/OR RESPIRATORY DISEASES

Patients with chronic cardiopulmonary disease (angina, heart failure, chronic obstructive pulmonary disease [COPD] and reactive airways disease) are often inactive and may be unable to follow recommendations to increase physical activity. Combining cardiopulmonary rehabilitation and exercise training may therefore help patients increase their daily energy expenditure and improve quality of life.

Weight gain and central adiposity independently contribute to increased risk for hypertension, dysglycemia, dyslipidemia, left-ventricular heart disease, ventricular dysfunction, coronary heart disease, congestive heart failure, arrhythmias, peripheral artery disease, deep vein thrombosis, pulmonary embolism, stroke, and sudden death. Consequently, impaired cardiovascular function is common in obese patients. Symptomatic cardiopulmonary disease affects a patient's lifestyle, and treatment may both dramatically improve their quality of life and motivate them to undertake lifestyle changes.

OBSTRUCTIVE SLEEP APNEA

Poor sleep and sleep deprivation increase blood cortisol levels and decrease serum leptin levels, leading to metabolic changes that promote weight gain and increase appetite. Obstructive sleep apnea (OSA), an important cause of sleep disruption, is highly prevalent among obese patients as obesity causes anatomic and functional alterations in the pharyngeal airway and central nervous system. A 10% increase in weight is associated with a six-fold increase in the risk of developing moderate to severe OSA.

OSA increases a patient's risk for cardiovascular complications such as hypertension, nocturnal arrhythmias, sudden death, etc. It may predispose to worsening obesity through sleep deprivation, daytime somnolence, and metabolic disruptions that limit a patient's ability to engage in physical activity and make the dietary changes needed for sustainable weight management.

> ▶ **Pearl:** Diagnosis and management of severe OSA may be a prerequisite for effective obesity management.

To diagnose OSA, the clinician must be aware of the spectrum of acute and chronic neurocognitive, psychiatric, and nonspecific symptoms it can cause, even when patients are unaware that their sleep is disturbed. The Berlin Questionnaire (widely available, as are other validated checklists and questionnaires) is a useful screening tool, though simple questions can also be used, such as, "If you were on vacation, sleeping seven or more hours per night, would you expect to feel well rested?" Other indicative symptoms are loud snoring, awakenings coupled with gasping for breath, frequent awakening during the night, abnormal daytime sleepiness or fatigue, morning headaches, limited attention and memory loss.

Polysomnography is the gold standard in diagnosing OSA and assessing the effects of treatment. Although not curative, nasal continuous positive airway pressure (CPAP) is the treatment of choice for most patients because it is non-invasive and technically efficacious. It is important to note that many patients find falling asleep with high CPAP pressures to be difficult. Those patients may find that using automated positive airway pressure (APAP) devices is more comfortable as they will deliver high pressures on demand rather than continuously. For patients with mild to moderate sleep apnea who are unable to tolerate CPAP, a dental device called the Thornton Adjustable Positioner (TAP) may be worth trying.

REDUCED PULMONARY FUNCTION

There is a clear association between dyspnea and obesity in both adults and children. Although cardiopulmonary fitness as assessed by maximal oxygen consumption is generally preserved in obese patients, exercise capacity is reduced because of the higher metabolic cost of carrying extra body weight. Obesity also increases the work involved in breathing because it reduces both chest wall compliance and respiratory muscle strength, which further contribute to the perception of increased breathing effort.

High BMI is typically associated with a reduction in forced expiratory volume in one second (FEV_1), forced vital capacity (FVC), total lung capacity, functional residual capacity, and expiratory reserve volume. Thoracic restriction associated with obesity is usually mild and is attributed to the mechanical effects of fat on the diaphragm and the chest wall: diaphragm excursion is impeded and thoracic compliance reduced. A clinically significant restrictive pattern (total lung capacity <85% predicted) is usually seen only in super-morbid obese patients (BMI >50) and hypercapnic respiratory failure and cor pulmonale are frequently observed in super-super-morbid obesity (BMI >60). Respiratory muscle strength may be compromised in obesity, and reduced maximal inspiratory pressure is often noted in obese patients.

When obesity is less than super-morbid, a restrictive defect should not be attributed to fat accumulation until other causes of restrictive impairment, such as interstitial lung disease or neuromuscular disease, have been excluded.

Patients with obesity frequently report dyspnea and wheezing and are often treated for asthma without objective diagnostic confirmation through pulmonary function testing. An accurate diagnosis is important because dyspnea related to other mechanisms or diseases may require a different therapeutic strategy. The diagnosis of asthma or COPD in obese individuals requires confirmation with spirometry and should not be based solely on symptoms.

> ▸ **Pearl:** Presuming that dyspnea is a function of obesity can lead you to miss other important and potentially life-threatening co-morbid dyspneic conditions.

Interventions aimed at improving pulmonary function may enable patients to be more physically active.

GASTROINTESTINAL DISORDERS

Dental Status
Elevated BMI is related to poor dental health status. Obesity is associated with increased prevalence of periodontal disease, particularly in younger individuals. Assessment of dental status is particularly important in obese patients, as food selection is affected by the number of teeth and occluding pairs of posterior teeth the patient has. Dental problems can limit a person's ability to eat food with high-fibre content, such as cereals, fruits and vegetables, and may push them to consume energy-dense processed foods.

Reflux Disease
Obesity brings an increased risk of gastroesophageal reflux disease symptoms, erosive esophagitis, and esophageal adenocarcinoma. The risk for these disorders seems to increase with increasing weight. Obesity has been associated with increased intra-abdominal pressure, impaired gastric emptying, decreased lower esophageal sphincter pressure, and increased frequency of transient sphincter relaxation, all of which lead to increased esophageal acid exposure. Symptoms of reflux can be interpreted as hunger and are often relieved by eating. In this way, reflux can contribute to weight gain. There is some evidence to suggest that control of reflux disease can lead to weight loss.

> ▸ **Pearl:** In some patients, esophageal reflux contributes to weight gain as its symptoms are often interpreted as hunger, and because eating can relieve symptoms.

Constipation and Irritable Bowel Syndrome

Decreased mobility and a diet low in fibre may predispose obese patients to constipation. Chronic constipation, together with increased intra-abdominal pressure, can increase the risk of diverticular disease as well as the incidence of hemorrhoids. Obesity can also contribute to the development of inguinal and umbilical hernias as well as recurrent herniation following repair. Abdominal symptoms including bloating, flatulence and other objective or subjective gastrointestinal symptoms can lead patients to avoid certain foods, thereby limiting their ability to follow a healthy diet.

It is not uncommon for obese patients to blame their weight gain on constipation. Such patients should be asked about laxative abuse. Successful treatment of constipation has not been shown to produce any substantive weight loss.

ENDOCRINE DISORDERS

Diabetes Mellitus

Weight loss is particularly difficult for individuals with diabetes.

Individuals with type 1 diabetes are dependent on the exogenous administration of insulin, which may lead to weight gain or difficulty with weight loss.

Individuals with type 2 diabetes struggle with weight management for many reasons. Some, like those with type 1 diabetes, require exogenous insulin which can lead to weight gain. Others are treated with sulphonylureas or thiazolidinediones, both of which may also contribute iatrogenically to weight gain or impede weight loss. Patients with early stage 2 diabetes may be hyperinsulinemic, which can also impede weight-loss efforts. Insulin resistance is present in lean tissue but not in adipose tissue. The adipose tissue of someone with type 2 diabetes may therefore be exposed to very large amounts of daily insulin and, as a result, become more efficient at energy storage.

The drug of choice for those with type 2 diabetes who need to lose weight is the biguanide metformin, which does not contribute to weight gain and actually promotes weight loss. A possible explanation is that metformin decreases circulating insulin by increasing the body's insulin sensitivity and decreasing both hepatic gluconeogenesis and the gastrointestinal tract's absorption of glucose.

For type 2 diabetes patients who require insulin, only detemir insulin has been shown to be weight neutral.

In this group, glycemic control takes priority over weight management. Discontinuation of weight-contributing medications should not be part of a patient's management plan unless their glucose levels are under control.

Lifestyle measures can help achieve glycemic control. Patients should be advised to eat many small meals and snacks throughout the day, minimize their intake of refined carbohydrates, increase their intake of whole grains and protein, and undertake short bouts of exercise several times a day.

Weight loss and fitness independently improve glycemic control and decrease insulin resistance. In some cases, they can be sufficient to control type 2 diabetes.

Hypothyroidism

Although hypothyroidism is associated with some weight gain, in most obese patients thyroid hormones are within normal levels. Hypothyroidism is associated with fluid retention and decreased resting energy expenditure, which may also contribute to weight gain. A patient with hypothyroidism that is severe enough to cause weight gain will, in virtually all cases, also display the other symptoms of hypothyroidism.

> ▸ **Pearl:** Most of the weight gain in hypothyroidism is due to water retention, not increased body fat.

Routine testing of thyroid hormones should be discouraged. Only patients with symptoms suggesting hypothyroidism (such as dry hair and skin, cold intolerance, hair loss, difficulty concentrating, poor memory, constipation, muscle cramping, menorrhagia and/or goitre) should be investigated.

Cushing's Syndrome

Ruling out Cushing's syndrome in patients with obesity is a clinical challenge, as obesity is one of the hallmark features of the disorder. The classic fat distribution in Cushing's syndrome is central, without affecting the extremities. Many metabolic abnormalities (hypertension, diabetes, hirsutism, menstrual irregularities) are found in both obesity and Cushing's syndrome. Certain features characteristic of Cushing's syndrome (easy bruising, purple striae, skin atrophy, proximal myopathy, hypokalemia, etc.) should prompt further investigation. The differential diagnosis of obesity from Cushing's syndrome and pseudo-Cushing's syndrome is clinically important for therapeutic decisions.

Cortisol levels are used to diagnose Cushing's, but obesity alone often causes elevated morning cortisol levels. If Cushing's is suspected, 24-hour urinary cortisol is a more sensitive test.

Polycystic Ovary Syndrome

Polycystic ovary syndrome (PCOS) is the most common female endocrinopathy, affecting between 6% and 10% of premenopausal women. It is associated with a significantly higher likelihood of developing various cardiovascular risk factors. Many women with PCOS (between 38% and 88%) are overweight or obese.

The etiology of PCOS is complex and multifactorial. There is much evidence, however, to suggest that adipose tissue plays an important role in the development and maintenance of PCOS, which is often accompanied by hyperinsulinemia.

There is a close correlation between adiposity and symptom severity in women with PCOS, and even modest reductions in weight generally bring significant improvement in menstrual regularity, fertility, and hyperandrogenic features.

Treatment involves metformin to treat PCOS-related hyperinsulinemia, which can help reduce symptoms and restore regular menstrual cycles.

See page 50 for a more thorough overview of PCOS treatment.

> ▸ **Pearl:** An obese patient who is oligomenorrheic should be considered to have PCOS until proven otherwise, and should be investigated promptly.

Testosterone Deficiency

Low levels of total and free testosterone in men may result in increased body fat and decreased lean tissue. Testosterone treatment in hypogonadic men restores lean tissue distribution. Total serum testosterone is inversely correlated with weight. Testosterone and blood concentrations of sex hormone binding globulin (SHBG) progressively decrease in obese men, but free testosterone levels usually remain normal. Massively obese men may have decreased total and free testosterone levels due to an increased adipose-tissue-mediated peripheral conversion of androgens to estrogens.

Aging is accompanied by a gradual decrease in free testosterone levels and increase in body fat. The term andropause has been used to describe symptoms thought to be related to low levels of bioavailable testosterone, including decreased strength and endurance, fatigue, low libido, irritability, and erectile dysfunction.

Testosterone replacement is not currently an accepted or proven adjunct in weight management and its use should be restricted to the symptomatic relief of andropause.

Hypothalamic Disorders

Any disorder that involves damage to the hypothalamus can lead to marked obesity. The hypothalamus is the brain's appetite centre and also regulates a great number of hormones. Disruptions to hormone regulation can lead to weight gain. Hormones controlled by the hypothalamus include human growth hormone, prolactin, thyroid-stimulating hormone, adrenocorticotropic hormone and the gonadotropins luteinizing hormone and follicle-stimulating hormone.

In children and young adults, the most common cause of hypothalamic dysfunction is craniopharyngioma, which is often associated with hyperphagia and obesity. Treatment involves surgical resection.

Growth hormone deficiency usually presents in early childhood with increased abdominal adiposity, short stature and fasting hypoglycemia. In adults, it presents with increased abdominal adiposity, reduced strength and exercise capacity, cold intolerance and often other symptoms of panhypopituitarism. Traumatic brain injuries, subarachnoid hemorrhage, and cerebrovascular accidents can also lead to hypothalamic dysfunction. Recombinant human growth hormone can be used to treat growth hormone deficiency.

[CHAPTER 6: LIFESTYLE ASSESSMENT]

The assessment of eating and physical activity patterns is an essential component of obesity management. The goal is to identify conditions and behaviours that may compromise treatment success.

EATING PATTERNS

A patient's eating patterns provide important clues about possible contributors to obesity and will help you design an appropriate treatment plan. Eating behaviour is highly variable. Some behaviours meet the stringent criteria of an eating disorder as defined by DSM-IV criteria (e.g., binge-eating disorder or bulimia). Other abnormal eating behaviours can be considered maladaptive rather than formally diagnosable. These include meal skipping, snack skipping, emotional eating, stress eating, boredom eating and night eating syndrome. Such behaviours are often not accompanied by feelings of guilt or distress.

Certain criteria need to be assessed to characterize different eating behaviours and address them in the treatment plan. Ask patients about the following:

1. Amount of food they eat during meals and snacks
2. Context (e.g., alone, special occasions, restaurants, time of day)
3. Hunger/cravings/compulsions
4. Satiety
5. Satiation
6. Fullness
7. Rate of eating
8. Physical state (e.g., tired, alert)
9. Energy intake
10. Macronutrient composition of diet
11. Emotional experience surrounding eating by assessing
    a. cognitive stimuli
    b. affective stimuli
    c. experience or lack of experience of loss of control
    d. feelings before (e.g., anger, loneliness), during (e.g., "numbing out," shame), and after (e.g., disgust, calmness)
12. Eating in the absence of physical hunger
13. Eating following overly aggressive restrictive diets or fasting
14. Eating after ingesting a food that heretofore they had been avoiding as part of a restrictive diet

Source: **Tanosky-Kraff, et al.** Eating disorder or disordered eating? Nonnormative eating patterns in obese individuals. *Obesity Research* 12:1361-1366 (2004).

Specific issues about eating patterns are addressed on the following pages.

Hunger and Disorganized Eating

Most patients and clinicians think of hunger as the physical pangs felt in the vicinity of the stomach (growling, moving, gurgling, constricting) combined with a desire to eat. We refer to this as physical or homeostatic hunger.

Many patients will deny that they ever feel physical hunger, and yet they find themselves eating in a manner that is inconsistent with their weight-management goals. These patients often refer to themselves as "emotional eaters" or "stress eaters" and commonly blame their lack of dietary control on abstract factors such as willpower, stress, depression, anxiety, boredom, and habit.

Emotional eating is the practice of consuming comfort foods or junk foods in response to feelings other than physical hunger. This can best be described as emotional or hedonistic hunger. We can call it *appetite*.

Emotional eating has a partially biological basis in that it appears to involve serotonin-releasing brain neurons — and the release of serotonin is controlled by food intake. Carbohydrate consumption in particular leads to the secretion of insulin, and the resultant insulin-mediated change in the body's plasma tryptophan ratio increases the release of serotonin. Protein intake does not stimulate insulin production and consequently does not produce the same effect. Because serotonin release is also involved in functions such as falling asleep, sensitivity to pain, blood pressure regulation, and mood control, many patients learn to overeat carbohydrates (particularly snack foods like potato chips or pastries, which are rich in both carbohydrates and fats) to make themselves feel better. Such patients are, in effect, self-medicating with food. This tendency appears in patients who gain weight during stressful periods of life, in women with severe premenstrual syndrome, in patients with SAD or depression, and in patients who are trying to stop smoking. (Nicotine, like dietary carbohydrates, increases brain serotonin secretion, while nicotine withdrawal decreases it.)

Other central neurotransmitters like the endocannabinoid system and the dopaminergic system may also be involved in the impulse to ingest certain foods to improve mood or alleviate physical symptoms.

Interestingly, most patients report having a time of day at which they find it most challenging to maintain dietary control, and other times of day at which they have no difficulties whatsoever.

Based on anecdotal evidence from many patients, we wonder whether emotional eaters should be divided into primary and secondary sub-groups. The majority of self-proclaimed emotional eaters would fall into the secondary sub-group, who only tend to eat emotionally from mid-afternoon onwards. While these individuals may have a heightened physiologic response to carbohydrates and use food to self-medicate, the fact that they do not struggle with emotional eating in the mornings suggests that some other factor is needed to trigger their eating behaviours. Many of these secondary emotional eaters admit to skipping or having very light breakfasts, no mid-morning snack, and sometimes light lunches. We wonder whether or not it is possible that these secondary emotional eaters require the combination of an emotion with a physiologic mechanism such as increased ghrelin, generated as a result of their disordered eating patterns that combine synergistically to trigger binge behaviours.

Given the incredibly important role of eating in the evolutionary development of every organism, we are tempted to expand the definition of hunger to include not only overt physical symptoms, but also appetite-mediated food cravings and food compulsiveness that trigger behaviours such as binge eating, emotional eating, and night eating in predisposed individuals. These behaviours often involve a loss of restraint, and individuals with a predisposition to this type of temporal disinhibition may be manifesting heritable mechanisms that evolved to allow for excess intake during times when food was only intermittently available.

Primary emotional eaters, on the other hand, self-medicate with food all day long in response to emotions and stressors. Rarer than secondary emotional eaters, these individuals are often much more difficult to treat and may well benefit from counselling from a clinical psychologist.

Mindless Eating

Brian Wansink coined the term "mindless eating" to describe hidden cues that trigger eating behaviours, such as family, friends, packaging, plate size, names and numbers, labels, colours, shapes, smells, distractions, distances, cupboards, and containers. It is possible that response to these cues also has roots in evolutionary biology.

One cue in particular may play a significant role in your patients' difficulties with weight management: social eating. Put simply, the more people we eat with, the more we tend to eat. This may result from being encouraged by others to eat, or eating to fit in, but sometimes, as Dr. Wansink suggests, it is completely mindless. Consider how this might influence your patient's weight if he or she has a wine-and-dine sales job, multiple work meetings or a circle of friends or family who centre all of their social interactions on food.

EXERCISE AND ACTIVITY

Exercise is an important determinant of health, and has beneficial effects on aerobic fitness, insulin sensitivity, blood pressure and coronary heart disease risk reduction, regardless of a patient's weight. It is also an important factor in weight management.

Asking patients about the type and amount of physical activity they undertake on a daily basis provides clues about the amount of energy they expend. It is important to explore types of activity undertaken at work and during leisure time. Patients may describe themselves as extremely busy and active at work, but careful questioning may reveal that they are in fact running to and from the car, to and from the elevator, and to and from their desk. While busy, they are not really physically active at levels sufficient to elicit an exercise response.

Different occupations involve different levels of activity, but in our day and age, it is exceedingly rare for a patient to be very physically active at work. Even occupations that were traditionally quite strenuous, such as farming, have incorporated labour- and time-saving devices that increase productivity while diminishing the farmer's expenditure of physical energy.

One way to obtain an objective measurement of activity is using a pedometer. Patients may talk of targeting 10,000 steps in their weight-management program, but a target set too far above what the patient is accustomed to is much less likely to be met. Establish a baseline and work from there to gradually increase activity levels.

Patients will often complain they do not have time for physical activity. It is important to explain that, from a weight-management perspective, exercise is cumulative and they do not need to find an hour every day to devote exclusively to physical fitness. Every 10 minutes of exercise counts, and virtually everything counts as exercise: walking, gardening, house work, playing with children, etc. Only a small minority of patients can motivate themselves to visit a gym on a regular basis, but most can find multiple 10-minute blocks of increased activity a day.

If patients have exercise equipment in their homes, encourage them to move the treadmill or stationary bicycle from the basement to the living room where it can better assert its existence.

Patients can be taught to establish cues that will help them remember to exercise. For example, to watch a favourite television program, they must be at least walking on the treadmill. Reward systems work too: for every 'x' minutes of exercise, the patient allows him- or herself some form of non-food-based reward.

Explain to patients that the calories they burn through exercise on a daily basis are not significant enough to warrant extra foods or increased portion sizes. People dramatically overestimate the calories burned through exercise, so remind them that the calories burned in 30 minutes of intense exercise can be consumed in 30 seconds with an increased portion size or a simple chocolate bar. However, over time, exercise can have a dramatic impact on weight and can greatly reduce the risk of regaining lost weight.

> ▶ **Pearl:** Exercise is not a license to overeat, but if a patient is exercising for more than 45 minutes at a stretch, they should be advised to fuel themselves before exercise with about 150 carbohydrate-based calories to minimize post-exercise hunger and provide their muscles with adequate energy.

[CHAPTER 7: CLINICAL ASSESSMENT]

Obesity affects virtually every organ system, and a comprehensive history and physical exam is an essential first step to treatment. Chapter 1 outlined the prerequisites for office set-up, for putting obese patients at ease during the clinical encounter. Body size can make physical examination difficult, reducing the clinical sensitivity of palpation, percussion, and auscultation. Severely obese patients may take longer to undress and may need assistance putting their clothes and shoes back on. Excessive sweating and limited physical hygiene due to difficulty in reaching all parts of the body may pose further embarrassment. Simple requests such as providing a urine or stool sample may be physically impossible for patients who cannot access their private parts. Clinical assessment includes determining the patient's degree of obesity, which affects their risk of co-morbidities. A number of tools can be used in combination to avoid some of the shortcomings each method has on its own.

BODY SIZE, SHAPE AND COMPOSITION

Table 6: Classification of obesity and waist circumference (WC) cut-offs			
	BMI (kg/m²)	Obesity Class	Risk of co-morbidities
Underweight	<18.5		Low
Normal	18.5–24.9		Average
Overweight	25–29.9		Mildly increased
Obesity	30–34.9	Class I	Moderate
	35–39.9	Class II	Severe
	>40	Class III	Very severe
Source: Adapted from the World Health Organization.			

BMI, calculated by dividing weight in kilograms by height in metres squared, provides a good measure of weight-related statistical risk of co-morbidities in population-based studies. On an individual level, however, the usefulness of BMI in ascertaining risk decreases as the body composition of people with similar BMIs can vary widely, especially at lower weights. For example, an athlete with a BMI of 32 and 15% body fat clearly does not have an indication for obesity treatment and likely faces minimal or no weight-related medical risk. On the other hand, a sedentary individual with a BMI of 27 and 30% body fat is likely at increased weight-related risk for co-morbidities. While easy to measure and entirely reproducible, BMI fails to take into account differences in race, sex, body frame, musculature, and age, all of which affect the ability to ascribe risk on an individual basis.

Other methods of assessing body composition include electrical bio-impedance analysis (BIA), dual X-ray absorptiometry (DEXA) and air-displacement plethysmography (BodPod®). While DEXA is the more accurate measure, repeated tests are expensive and expose patients to radiation. In contrast, BIA is cheap and accessible and, despite its imprecision (measures vary dramatically with the patient's level of hydration), is often used by weight-management centres to monitor changes in body composition during weight loss. While the diagnostic and prognostic utility of measuring body composition remains debatable, some clinicians find it helpful for counselling and motivating select patients. The risk with BIA is that body fat percentage changes quite slowly and, coupled with the inaccuracy of office BIA analysis, this can mean that body fat percentage measurements can change barely from one visit to the next. The patient who has lost a medically significant amount of weight may find this discouraging.

> **Pearl:** While the target in weight management should be a patient's best weight, all patients have a number target in mind. If they find themselves discouraged by a less-than-target amount of weight loss, you can try reframing the result as a percentage of both the target they have in their heads, and of their best weight target.
>
> Example: Your patient wants to lose 18 kg (40 lbs) and has lost 11 kg (25 lbs) and feels discouraged. Reframe this by telling them they have achieved over 60% of their weight-loss target.

More important than the absolute amount of body fat is its location. Intra-abdominal or visceral adipose tissue is a better predictor than BMI of cardio-metabolic risk factors, respiratory impairment, fatty liver, and reflux disease. The easiest way to assess abdominal adiposity in clinical practice is by measuring waist circumference. This is best done by positioning the patient in front of the seated examiner, identifying the bony landmark (upper edge of the iliac crest), and asking the patient to hold onto the tape and turn around, thereby bringing the tape around the abdomen. After ensuring that the tape is snug and parallel to the ground, the circumference is measured at the end of a regular expiration using the cross-arm technique. Table 7 on page 43 details the waist circumference cut-offs for identifying central obesity for different ethnic groups.

Table 7: Waist circumference as measure of central obesity (pragmatic cut-offs)	
Ethnic Group	**Waist circumference (cm)**
Europids / Sub-Saharan Africans / Eastern Mediterranean and Middle East/Arab	
Men	>94 cm
Women	>80 cm
South Asians / Ethnic South and Central Americans	
Men	>90 cm
Women	>80 cm
Chinese Men	>90 cm
Women	>80 cm
Japanese Men	>85 cm
Women	>90 cm

Source: **Alberti, K.G.M.M. et al.** The metabolic syndrome – a new worldwide definition. *The Lancet*; 1059-1062: 366 2005.

> ▸ **Pearl**: Waist circumference measurements add little to risk stratification in patients with BMIs >40.

EDMONTON OBESITY STAGING SYSTEM

Although higher BMI levels are generally associated with greater mental, medical and functional problems, anthropometric measures alone are not a good reflection of the severity or extent of obesity-related co-morbidities. Sharma and Kushner have recently suggested a clinical staging system to complement the BMI when describing the severity of obesity.

The Edmonton Obesity Staging System consists of the following five stages:

Stage 0: Patient has no apparent obesity-related risk factors (e.g., blood pressure, serum lipids, fasting glucose, etc. within normal range), no physical symptoms, no psychopathology, no functional limitations or impairment of well-being.

Stage 1: Patient has one or more obesity-related sub-clinical risk factors (e.g., elevated blood pressure, impaired fasting glucose, elevated liver enzymes, etc.), mild physical symptoms (e.g., dyspnea on moderate exertion, occasional aches and pains, fatigue, etc.), mild psychopathology, mild functional limitations and/or mild impairment of well-being.

Stage 2: Patient has one or more established obesity-related chronic diseases requiring medical treatment (e.g., hypertension, type 2 diabetes, sleep apnea, osteoarthritis, reflux disease, polycystic ovary syndrome, anxiety disorder, etc.), moderate functional limitations and/or moderate impairment of well-being.

Stage 3: Patient has clinically significant end-organ damage such as myocardial infarction, heart failure, diabetic complications, incapacitating osteoarthritis, significant psychopathology, significant functional limitations and/or significant impairment of well-being.

Stage 4: Patient has severe (potentially end-stage) disabilities from obesity-related chronic diseases, severe disabling psychopathology, severe functional limitations and/ or severe impairment of well-being

The Edmonton Obesity Staging System is used together with BMI class as follows:

Case 1: A 24-year-old physically active female with a BMI of 32 kg/m² with no demonstrable risk factors, functional limitations or self-esteem issues would have Class I, Stage 0 Obesity. In this patient the focus would be on prevention of further weight gain. Health benefits of more aggressive obesity treatment would likely be marginal.

Case 2: A 32-year-old male with a BMI of 36 kg/m² who also has essential hypertension and obstructive sleep apnea would have Class II, Stage 2 Obesity. This person would have a clear indication for obesity treatment.

Case 3: A 45-year-old female with BMI of 54 kg/m² who is in a wheelchair because of disabling arthritis and severe hypopnea would have Class III, Stage 4 Obesity. This patient will either require aggressive obesity treatment or be deemed palliative.

METABOLISM

People often talk about their extra weight as a consequence of having a "slow metabolism." In this context, metabolism refers to total daily energy expenditure and is made up of three components: basal metabolic rate (BMR), which is the energy spent on basal metabolism, energy spent on physical activity, and increases in resting energy expenditure in response to different stimuli such as thermogenesis or the thermic effect of food.

BMR is, for most people, the largest component of energy expenditure. It typically accounts for between 60% and 75% of total daily energy expenditure. BMR can be measured through indirect analysis of the amount of heat produced by an individual, using the amount of oxygen consumed and the Weir equations. This means of analysis is called indirect calorimetry and is the current gold standard in office-based BMR measurement. Ideally, it should be measured under standardized conditions, with the patient awake, lying in the supine position, in a resting state in a comfortable warm environment, in the morning, and 10-12 hours after the last meal. In many weight management practices, strict adherence to these conditions is often overlooked. Testing involves connecting the patient to an indirect calorimeter, which measures how much oxygen is inspired and expired during the test. Most tests take 20 minutes to complete. By far the most important determinant of BMR is body size, in particular fat-free (lean) body mass. Even then, BMR can vary by up to 10% in individuals of the same age, gender, body size, and fat-free mass, suggesting that genetic or other factors are also involved.

Patients often overlook the fact that as they lose weight, they lose not only fat but also fat-free mass, as their muscles adapt to the lighter workload after carrying around extra weight. With enough weight loss, BMR tends to decrease. In addition, hormonal and metabolic responses to weight loss will further reduce energy requirements. Progressive weight loss means people will need fewer and fewer calories because their total daily energy expenditure has decreased.

NUTRITIONAL STATUS

Despite a high caloric intake, obese patients often have a number of dietary deficiencies in both macro- and micro-nutrients. Overall nutritional intake is best assessed using food diaries or food frequency questionnaires. While these tools provide a good picture of eating patterns, they do not usually provide an accurate assessment of actual caloric intake unless patients are explicitly taught how to keep them. Food recall is notoriously inaccurate and most patients significantly underestimate true portion sizes.

- Inadequate protein intake can reduce satiety and promote the loss of lean body mass.
- Inadequate intake of complex carbohydrates can lead to B-vitamin deficiencies.
- Inadequate intake of fruits and vegetables can lead to deficiencies in folic acid, magnesium and other minerals.
- Inadequate intake of dairy products, together with decreased exposure to sunlight, can result in clinically significant calcium and vitamin D deficiencies, resulting in secondary hyperparathyroidism and loss of bone mineral mass.
- Avoidance of red meat can result in iron deficiencies in women.
- Nutritional deficiencies are particularly common in people adhering to fad diets, individuals from lower-income strata, and following bariatric surgery.

Although physical signs of nutritional deficiency are not commonly found, the presence of hair loss, easily plucked hair, spooning of the nails, glossitis and or cheilosis, should prompt the evaluation of mineral and vitamin deficiencies.

> ▸ **Pearl:** Nutritional deficiencies (Vitamins D, B12, folate, iron, etc.) are common in obese patients.

CARDIO-CIRCULATORY SYSTEM

Abdominal obesity is now widely recognized as being an independent risk factor for cardiovascular disease, as it promotes hypertension as well as glucose and lipid abnormalities, all of which increase cardiovascular risk. It is therefore not surprising that obesity is often associated with high blood pressure, ischemic heart disease, stroke, type 2 diabetes, and dyslipidemia. Obesity has also been associated with several non-traditional risk factors, such as disturbance of fibrinolysis, impaired endothelial function, and chronic low-grade inflammation. It is interesting that a significant subset of obese patients appear to be metabolically healthy, and the assumption is that their expanded subcutaneous adipose tissue acts as a "metabolic sink" and protects them from the cardio-metabolic consequences of obesity.

Obesity is associated with left ventricular hypertrophy that is not just related to concomitant hypertension. Increases in stroke volume, cardiac output, and diastolic dysfunction are seen in obese patients even without hypertension. The right ventricle also changes as a result of left ventricular dysfunction or the coexistence of obstructive sleep apnea or hypoventilation syndrome. For all of these reasons, heart failure in obesity is generally biventricular.

Obesity is not only related to hemodynamic and structural changes in the heart, but it can also predispose to arrhythmias and might be a predisposing factor for sudden death. Risk factors for obesity-related arrhythmias include left ventricular hypertrophy, congestive heart failure, autonomic imbalance, and sleep apnea.

Obesity contributes to chronic venous stasis disease of the lower extremities, as it increases abdominal pressure and leads to impaired venous and lymphatic return. Morbidly obese patients are at increased risk for edema and lymphedema in the lower extremities, stasis ulcers, thrombophlebitis, deep venous thrombosis and pulmonary thromboembolism.

Unfortunately, morbidly obese patients are less likely to receive appropriate diagnosis and treatment as adequate diagnostic equipment for these patients is not always available. Most cardiac diagnostic equipment is not suitable for patients who weigh more than 181.5 kg (400 lbs).

It is important to identify obese patients who are particularly at risk for cardiovascular complications. History and physical exam should address symptoms and signs of organ damage (coronary artery disease, peripheral vascular disease, congestive heart failure) and diagnostic procedures should be performed where indicated. It is also important to recognize that cardiovascular problems such as angina, exertional dyspnea and intermittent claudication can promote weight gain by making exercise more difficult and potentially risky. Reduced capacity for physical activity is particularly relevant in patients who have suffered paralytic strokes.

You should ascertain a patient's family history of diabetes and premature cardiovascular disease as well as their physical activity status. As well, the following risk factors for cardiovascular disease should be thoroughly explored in all obese patients.

Dysglycemia
Patients who develop type 2 diabetes experience a progressive deterioration of glucose tolerance over time, from normoglycemia to impaired fasting glucose or impaired glucose tolerance, to overt diabetes. Most patients with type 2 diabetes are obese, and abdominal obesity has been recognized as a significant risk factor for the development of type 2 diabetes. With the exception of metformin, the pharmacological treatment of diabetes generally promotes weight gain. This includes sulphonylureas, thiazolidinediones, and most insulins. Newer hypoglycemic agents including insulins (e.g., detemir), long-acting insulin analogues (e.g., insulin, glargine, detemir), and DPP-IV inhibitors (e.g., sitagliptin, vildagliptin) may have a lower risk for weight gain. A new class of GLP-1 agonists (e.g., exenatide, liraglutide) may induce modest weight loss.

> ▸ **Pearl:** When ordering blood tests, include fasting glucose, HbA1c and fasting insulin: Early in the progression of type 2 diabetes, one might expect to see hyperinsulinemia in the absence of hyperglycemia or changes in HbA1c. This finding should make you more vigilant in your surveillance and may provide your patient with increased motivation for initiating a weight-management effort.

Dyslipidemia

Obesity-associated dyslipidemia has been shown to be atherogenic. Abdominal obesity is associated with increases in plasma triglycerides and decreases in HDL cholesterol. The effect of obesity on LDL cholesterol is less clear, but obese individuals have increased atherogenic small, dense LDL particles and elevated levels of apolipoprotein B (Apo B). Increased levels of lipoprotein a (Lpa) are also commonly seen in patients with abdominal obesity.

Hypertension

Hypertension is closely related to abdominal obesity, particularly in younger individuals. Obesity-related hypertension is characterized by sodium retention, increased sympathetic activity and activation of the renin-angiotensin-aldosterone system (RAAS).

Obstructive Sleep Apnea

The presence of obstructive sleep apnea is an important cause of "resistant" hypertension in obese patients and should be formally ruled out in all obese hypertensive patients. Screening for sleep apnea is covered in Chapter 5.

Smoking Status

Smoking cessation is a major goal for cardiopulmonary risk management. It is important to recognize that smoking is commonly used as a weight-control measure, particularly in younger women. The fear of weight gain should be acknowledged as a significant obstacle to smoking cessation, but it is less likely to produce negative health consequences than continued smoking.

ENDOCRINE SYSTEM

Although they are rare, we need to be careful not to miss endocrinal causes of obesity. These include hypothyroidism and Cushing's syndrome (see page 35), as well as growth-hormone and testosterone deficiencies.

> ▸ **Pearl:** It is exceedingly rare for a patient to have an endocrinal cause of obesity that is not accompanied by other signs and symptoms. Biochemical exploration for these conditions is therefore not recommended unless additional clinical signs or symptoms suggest the presence of these disorders.

For some patients, knowing there is no endocrinal cause for their obesity can remove a psychological barrier to adopting a weight management effort.

While an increasing number of hormone-like substances released from various organs (leptin from adipose tissue, ghrelin from the stomach, PYY 3-36 from the colon) are recognized as playing an important role in the regulation of energy balance, diagnostic tests for disorders involving these novel hormones have not yet found their way into clinical practice, nor are there therapies available to address these specific contributors.

DIGESTIVE SYSTEM

Obesity increases the risk of gallbladder disease, particularly in women. Cholesterol gallstones are most common and are the only type of calculi with a clear relationship to obesity. Potential causes of increased gallstone formation in obesity include changes in bile composition and gallbladder emptying.

Gallstone formation increases significantly during periods of rapid weight loss. Patients who have lost weight rapidly in the past are at increased risk for gallstone disease.

Very low-calorie diets and bariatric surgery both dramatically increase the risk of symptomatic gallstone disease, most likely as a consequence of reduced gallbladder emptying and motility. Some surgeons advocate routine cholecystectomy during bariatric surgery, but this remains controversial as it may increase the chance of surgical complications. In patients with gallstones or sludge, prophylaxis with ursodeoxycholic acid 500 mg twice daily may help to reduce the risk of symptomatic gallstone disease and can be used during periods of rapid weight loss.

Non-alcoholic fatty liver disease (NAFLD) is an increasingly recognized condition that can progress to end-stage liver disease. NAFLD refers to a wide spectrum of liver damage, ranging from simple steatosis (excessive hepatic lipid accumulation) to steatohepatitis, advanced fibrosis and cirrhosis. Simple steatosis may have the best prognosis within the spectrum, but it can progress to steatohepatitis, fibrosis and even cirrhosis. Insulin resistance and oxidative stress play critical roles in the pathogenesis of non-alcoholic fatty liver disease.

Steatosis is found in two-thirds of obese patients and more than 90% of morbidly obese patients. Both the presence and severity of steatosis correlate positively with adiposity. Truncal obesity seems to be an important risk factor even in patients with a normal BMI. Steatohepatitis affects around 20% of obese and almost 50% of morbidly obese populations. Steatohepatitis has been found even in children under the age of 10, and may become more common with the current explosion in childhood obesity rates.

Most patients with non-alcoholic liver disease have no symptoms or signs of liver disease at the time of diagnosis, though some report generalized fatigue or malaise. NAFLD is characterized by hepatomegaly and mild to moderate elevations in serum transaminase levels (specifically ALT with the ALT:AST ratio usually <1). The presence of hypoalbuminemia, prolonged PT and hyperbilirubinemia are much more worrisome and suggest progression toward cirrhosis. Ultrasonography and computer-assisted tomography can detect the fatty infiltration of the liver, but liver biopsy remains the most sensitive and specific means of determining the presence of inflammation and fibrosis, thus providing important prognostic information.

NEUROLOGICAL ISSUES

Pseudotumour cerebri is a syndrome involving raised intracranial pressure without clinical, laboratory or radiological evidence of intracranial pathology. It is usually seen in young obese women. Long a relatively rare disease, incidence is growing rapidly along with increasing rates of obesity. The cause is unknown but it is thought to be related to increased intracranial pressure that produces symptoms such as headache, nausea, vomiting and pulsatile tinnitus. Permanent visual defects are serious and not infrequent complications. Weight loss can usually reverse symptoms of pseudotumour cerebri and prevent the onset of permanent complications. Fundoscopic examination of patients with pseudotumour cerebri may reveal what appears to be papilledema.

RENAL ISSUES

Obesity is associated with renal risk factors such as hypertension and diabetes, but also with an unfavourable renal hemodynamic profile. This results in both functional (sodium retention, mircroalbuminuria) and morphological (glomerulomegaly, focal segmental glomerulosclerosis) changes that can sometimes produce a progressive fall in glomerular filtration rate and a further rise in urinary albumin excretion. Together, these can lead to the development of proteinuria, and, in rare cases, end-stage renal failure.

In patients with end-stage renal failure, severe obesity may pose a problem for vascular access, and complicate peritoneal dialysis and renal transplantation.

Obesity is also associated with an increased risk for kidney stones and renal cancer.

Excess weight is a recognized risk factor for urinary stress incontinence.

REPRODUCTIVE SYSTEM

Patients with morbid obesity report a decrease in desire, less enjoyment from sexual activity, difficulty with sexual performance and avoidance of sexual encounters.

Overweight and obese women have an increased incidence of dysfunctional uterine bleeding and amenorrhea. Elevated plasma testosterone and androstenedione are frequently found alongside reduced sex hormone binding globulin (SHBG) and increased ratio of estrone to estradiol. The obesity-related increase in androgen production evident in obese women may be due to an increase in ovarian and adrenal production stimulated by insulin, and a consequent reduction in SHBG. Adipose tissue may have a peripheral effect on steroid secretion and serve as a reservoir and site for steroid generation.

Massively obese men may have subnormal plasma testosterone concentrations and reduced SHBG levels. Low levels of testosterone and growth hormone have been associated with increased deposition of abdominal fat. The inverse relationship between plasma testosterone and body weight in obese men may be attributable to increased aromatization of androgen precursors to estrogens by adipose tissue, resulting in negative feedback on the hypothalamic-pituitary axis. It is important to note that there is currently no evidence to support the use of testosterone replacement in the treatment of obesity.

PCOS affects one in 10 women and is even more common in the obese population. The strong association between excess weight and PCOS raises the possibility that either obesity is a causal factor for PCOS, or PCOS is a causal factor for obesity. PCOS decreases fertility and is associated with a range of metabolic abnormalities including:
• Insulin resistance/hyperinsulinemia/impaired glucose tolerance/type 2 diabetes
• Dyslipidemia
• Increased estrone:estradiol ratio
• Decreased SHBG
• Increased free steroid concentrations

Symptoms of PCOS may include:
• Oligomenorrhea
• Infertility
• Hirsutism
• Acne, oily skin or dandruff
• Abdominal obesity
• Male pattern baldness
• Skin tags

Treatment of PCOS aims to alleviate symptoms. Oral contraceptives can help to restore regular menses, decrease ovarian testosterone secretion, and clear facial acne. Metformin can improve insulin sensitivity, thereby reducing insulin production and decreasing adrenal androgen production. Metformin can also help restore regular ovulation, decrease abnormal hair growth, reduce body weight, and improve dyslipidemia.

Weight loss is perhaps the best treatment for PCOS, and a 10% weight loss may be sufficient to restore normal ovulation and fertility.

SKIN PROBLEMS

Obesity is associated with a number of dermatoses. It affects cutaneous sensation, temperature regulation, foot shape, and vasculature.

Acanthosis nigricans is the most common dermatological manifestation of obesity and it appears as velvety, light brown-to-black markings usually on the neck, under the arms, or in the groin. Skin tags are more commonly associated with diabetes than with obesity, but may be an early clue to the presence of hyperinsulinemia.

Obesity increases the incidence of cutaneous infections such as candidiasis, intertrigo, candida folliculitis, furunculosis, erythrasma, tinea cruris, and folliculitis. Less common infections include cellulitis, necrotizing fasciitis, and gas gangrene.

Leg ulcerations, lymphedema, plantar hyperkeratosis, and striae are all more common with obesity.

Contrary to popular belief, cellulite is not related to obesity. It is part of normal female physiology and is present to some extent in over 95% of all adult women.

> ▶ **Pearl:** Lipidema, the edema secondary to lymphatic obstruction due to increased tissue pressure from fat accumulation, must be differentiated from lymphedema from other causes.

CANCER

There is a large and growing body of epidemiologic evidence supporting a causal relationship between obesity and cancer. Obesity is thought to account for 7.7% of all cancer diagnoses in Canada and being obese dramatically increases cancer-related mortality. To date, being overweight and obesity have been strongly associated with increased risks for esophageal, colorectal, gallbladder, pancreatic, breast, renal, uterine, cervical, and prostate cancers.

While there may be a clear relationship between obesity and cancer incidence, the mechanisms through which obesity predisposes to cancer are far less clear. In women, one possible mechanism involves the higher levels of free circulating estrogen commonly associated with obesity that result from both increased production in adipose tissue and decreased sex hormone binding protein (SHBP).

Central obesity is associated with high levels of insulin-like growth factor I (IGF-I), which inhibits apoptosis and stimulates cell proliferation. IGF-I is associated with diverse types of cancer (breast, ovarian, colorectal, lung, prostate and bladder).

[CHAPTER 8: TREATMENT]

> ▸ **Pearl:** In obesity treatment, one size does not fit all!

Obesity is a heterogeneous condition, and no single management strategy will work for all patients. As we have pointed out, there is currently no cure for obesity. Any successful management plan involves long-term coping strategies that help patients reduce their body weight and prevent weight regain. Treatment is typically characterized by intermittent periods of remission and relapse, commonly referred to as "weight cycling." The impact of weight cycling on obesity-related health risks remains controversial, but there is evidence to suggest that weight cycling results in increased body fat and makes subsequent weight-loss efforts more difficult.

Treatment goals must be realistic and focus on improving health status and quality of life, rather than just reducing a number on the scale. As discussed in Chapter 2, the goal you promote should be a patient's *best weight:* the healthiest lifestyle a patient can realistically enjoy, not the healthiest lifestyle a patient can tolerate. Goals expressed as a particular number of kilograms or percentage of body weight can lead patients to regard even weight losses that bring significant medical benefits as dramatic failures. Remember, health benefits can be achieved with as little as a 5%–10% weight loss. It is also important to remember that weight maintenance is just as important — if not more important — than weight loss in reducing health risks. The establishment of realistically achievable goals using the concept of best weight will help patients accept the effort involved in weight management.

Treatment strategies have traditionally described two distinct phases in obesity management: the *weight-loss* phase and the *weight-maintenance* phase. This may not, in fact, be the wisest approach. Unless a patient persists with the strategies they implement to achieve weight loss, they are likely to regain their weight, especially where these strategies focus on lifestyle. Lifestyle change is extremely difficult, and suggesting that a patient will need to implement two different sets of lifestyle strategies — first to lose weight and then to maintain weight loss — makes the program less sustainable.

If you can ensure that your patients are comfortable and confident with the lifestyle they adopt to lose weight, they are likely to persist with that lifestyle to maintain weight loss.

> ▸ **Pearl:** Regardless of the strategy your patient chooses for weight loss, unless they are able to confidently say that they could "live like this forever," they are likely to regain the weight.

In general, weight loss requires caloric restriction. A negative energy balance of about 500 kcal per day results in weight loss of about 1 to 2 kg (2 to 4 lbs) per month. A kilogram of fat tissue is equivalent to ~7000 kcal (3500 kcal/lb).

Treatment strategies should be individualized to promote adherence and facilitate success. In most cases, some combination of lifestyle change, regular physical activity, medication and surgery will significantly increase the likelihood of weight-loss maintenance.

The next three chapters will look at the wide range of options available within the broad categories of lifestyle/behaviour, medication, and surgery.

LIFESTYLE AND BEHAVIOUR CHANGE

Lifestyle change is the cornerstone of weight management, whether it is undertaken alone or in combination with pharmacologic or surgical strategies. There is no getting around the fact that weight management depends on controlling what you eat. This chapter aims to go beyond an examination of what patients eat to look more intently at *why* they eat, how they eat, and what behavioural strategies can help them change patterns and habits that impede weight management.

HUNGER PREVENTION

For years, we have been taught to encourage patients to wait until they are hungry before they eat. We now know that this is patently terrible advice.

A simple example illustrates the point: When we go to a supermarket hungry, most of us will end up buying foods that are not on our list, and buying more food than we need. Hunger influences our decisions.

Preparing or sitting down to a meal when hungry is no different — except in this case the "shopping" is being done from our cupboards, refrigerators, serving dishes or, worse still from a weight perspective, a restaurant menu.

To put it simply, hunger trumps reason. Your patient might be highly intelligent and motivated, but if he or she is hungry when sitting down to eat, they will find it very difficult to make healthy low-calorie choices. People do not crave leafy green salads when they are hungry.

It is much easier to eat sensibly when you are not hungry. Healthy eating begins with a wholesome breakfast and wholesome, low-calorie, satiating snacks between meals.

> ▸ **Pearl:** Recommend that your patients practice pre-emptive eating. We recommend that patients eat every 2–3 hours to minimize the effects of both physical and mental hunger on their dietary choices.

The hunger produced by meal and snack skipping almost always begins between mid-afternoon and early evening, rather than at the time of the skipped meal or snack. Studies on both leptin and ghrelin, two hormones whose role in the development of hunger are well described, show that they tend to trigger hunger in the evening in response to calories missed in the morning. If we look to evolutionary biology for explanation, this delayed response may have allowed our ancestors to postpone hunting and food gathering until later on in the day when sub-Saharan temperatures were more moderate and predators less plentiful.

PROTEIN

A myriad of studies has shown that in adults protein is more satiating than carbohydrates and fats. As well, the consumption of protein alongside carbohydrates delays carbohydrate absorption and attenuates the body's insulin response.

Some medical professionals still worry about the effects of a high-protein diet on renal function, but this concern is unwarranted in patients with normal renal function.

The consumption of protein with every meal or snack can help weight management by increasing satiety and blunting the insulin surges associated with the consumption of sugars and refined carbohydrates. These surges can lead to increased hunger. Protein consumption may also improve glycemic control.

We recommend intake of at least 1 g/kg/day of high quality mixed dietary protein to maintain lean body mass and sustain other essential body functions. High-protein diets may also be easier to follow due to increased satiation, though long-term weight-loss maintenance has not been shown to be superior on high-protein diets than on other hypo-caloric diets.

CARBOHYDRATES

Ensure that your patients consume at least 100 g/day (400 kcal/day) of carbohydrates to prevent protein breakdown, muscle wasting and large shifts in fluid balance.

Complex, whole-grain carbohydrates and those high in fibre are associated with greater satiety, while refined carbohydrates produce rapid and dramatic physiologic insulin responses, which may explain their association with the development of insulin resistance and type 2 diabetes.

> ▸ **Pearl:** The body can only store 24–48 hours worth of carbohydrates for future use. It is stored in the form of glycogen, primarily in muscle tissue and the liver. The reason low-carb diets such as Atkins produce such dramatic weight loss in the first week is that glycogen is stored with around 4.5 kg (10 lbs) of water, and when glycogen stores are depleted, that water is liberated. This is also why, when patients stop their low-carb diets, they have a tendency to immediately gain back that 10 lbs as their glycogen stocks are restored.

FAT

A growing body of evidence suggests that particular types of fat, rather than the overall quantity of fat, contribute most to cardiovascular risk. While trans fats and saturated fats have been strongly linked to cardiovascular disease, the opposite is true for unsaturated fats, which appear to be cardioprotective.

From a weight perspective, reducing fat intake is desirable given its high energy density. However, the indiscriminate reduction of dietary fat has not been shown to have any dramatic long-term benefit on weight.

Given the sharply elevated cardiovascular risk associated with weight and its co-morbidities, we would caution against recommending a low-fat diet per se. Instead, we would recommend that patients aim to reduce trans fats and saturated fats as much as possible while still leading an enjoyable life. We would also encourage the preferential consumption of healthy fats found in fish, various plant oils, and nuts.

CALORIE AWARENESS

Calories are the currency of weight. In this day and age, calorie information is readily available — posted on the packaging of every product in the supermarket and even on the menus of fast food restaurants. There are whole books and websites dedicated exclusively to helping people count dietary calories.

The best analogy for dietary record-keeping is money: before buying something, it is important to know how much you have in the bank, how much you make a month and how much the item costs. Similarly, before eating something, it is useful to know how many calories you burn in a day, how many calories you have had that day and how many calories are in the foods you are considering. If you know those three things, and you are not hungry, then you can ask, "Is it worth the calories?" If you are hungry, it is always worth the calories, but if you are not, it is important to remember that the calories might still be worth it. Food brings us pleasure. We celebrate and comfort with food. If your patient feels that they cannot use food for pleasure, their weight-loss efforts will be short-lived.

A food diary is probably the easiest way to conduct a calorie audit, but for it to be useful as a long-term tool, the diary should never be used to pass judgment on a patient's efforts, assess whether they have been "good" or "bad," or calculate how much "room" they have left for dinner. A food diary should simply be used to provide guidance.

Two things matter — completeness and accuracy.

Completeness involves writing foods down throughout the day. Studies have consistently demonstrated that when relying on end-of-day recall, people tend to forget what they have eaten. The easiest way to protect against food amnesia is to make notes throughout the day. We recommend that patients not calculate calories immediately but rather take 15 minutes at the end of the day to do their calculations. Calorie calculation takes time, and during a busy workday most people will get frustrated if they need to refer to a calorie-tracking resource constantly. We also want to discourage patients from using their calorie count as a restrictive ceiling and going to bed hungry, rather than exceeding a targeted caloric intake. Such behaviour will almost certainly result in the abandonment of the weight-management effort.

Accuracy is also important. The human eye is very bad at weighing and measuring. We recommend that patients use scales, spoons, and measuring cups to accurately track their food intake. It is important to emphasize that these tools are meant to measure how much they ate, not to determine how much they are allowed to eat. The patient who begins to view the measuring cup as a dictator will likely get frustrated and quit.

While food diaries can be kept on paper, there are also many free online resources that can be found using a simple Google search for "food diary."

Once a patient starts to see where their calories come from, it becomes much easier for them to identify changes they can make and maintain over the long-term. It may also be useful for them to know simple caloric equivalents. Knowing that a low-fat bran muffin has more calories than a cheeseburger may help them decide that the muffin probably isn't worth its calories.

Liquid Calories

Some of the easiest sources of calories to control are liquids. Many patients do not realize how many calories they are consuming even in so-called "healthy" drinks. A glass of juice provides as many calories as a glass of sugared soda. A glass of wine provides almost double that amount. Encourage your patients to choose zero-calorie beverages.

> ▸ **Pearl:** Aspartame and sucralose have been found to be safe in every major study and meta-analysis performed to date. The same cannot be said of sugar.

EATING HYGIENE

A solid body of research (see Brian Wansink in particular) has irrefutably demonstrated the importance of cultivating good eating hygiene. Avoiding mindless snacking in front of the television and shopping in big box stores. Using smaller plates, cups and bowls, buying food in the smallest possible containers, and keeping high-calorie foods out of sight (or out of house), will all help a patient's weight-management effort.

SUPPLEMENTS AND REPLACEMENTS

The main benefit of meal replacements in a weight-management strategy lies in their convenience and ability to promote portion control. A partial meal replacement plan prescribes a low-calorie diet (>800 <1600 kcal/day) in which one or two meals a day are replaced by commercially available, calorie-reduced products that are vitamin- and mineral-fortified, and at least one meal involves regular food. Satiety can be enhanced by meal replacements fortified with protein.

A wide range of commercial meal replacement products is available. They come either as powders that are mixed with milk or other liquids, or as bars. Most meal replacement products provide 220–300 kcal/meal and are relatively high in protein (14–18 g) and low in fat. Unfortunately, most are also low in fibre. To qualify as a meal replacement, these products must provide 30% of the recommended daily allowance (RDA) of most vitamins and minerals. Thus, with two meal replacements per day, patients are meeting at least 60% of their daily nutritional needs.

Meal replacements provide built-in portion and calorie control and a composition that is dense in nutrients but low in calories. Meal replacements simplify food choices, are rapidly prepared, and can be consumed anywhere.

> ▸ **Pearl:** Advise patients to stock up on meal replacements in their home, office, and car for "emergencies."

While meal replacements can safely and effectively produce significant weight loss and improve weight-related risk factors and co-morbidities, they can only be used for long-term weight management if patients continue to use them over the long-term.

> ▸ **Pearl:** For people who do not eat breakfast, a liquid, protein-supplemented, meal replacement is a simple way to ensure adequate caloric and protein intake in the morning.

Protein Supplements

Though few patients will be inclined to replace a meal forever, many more are comfortable using food supplements such as protein bars to replace higher-calorie, less nutritive snacks. Given the tremendous consumer demand for lower-calorie, better-tasting products, these have become much more palatable in recent years. From drinks and puddings to bars and soy nuts, there is now a myriad of protein-supplemented, calorie-controlled snacks available.

Given that these products generally contain little to no sugar, are less than 200 kcal and are fortified with satiating protein, they can prove to be quite beneficial even for patients who do not want to adopt a formal meal replacement strategy.

LOW AND VERY LOW-CALORIE DIETS

Low and very low-calorie diets (LCDs and VLCDs) often use calorie-controlled, high-protein, vitamin- and mineral- fortified liquid meals as the sole nutrient source (e.g., OPTIFAST 900). These diets provide between 1200 and 800 kcal/day (LCD) or less than 800 kcal/day (VLCD). They are typically used for 12–16 weeks to induce rapid weight loss. LCDs or VLCDs are sometimes prescribed for the super-morbidly obese or when rapid weight loss is an urgent medical necessity. Medical contraindications include pregnancy, type 1 diabetes, cardiovascular disease, cardiac conduction disorder, renal or hepatic disease, eating disorders, and acute psychiatric illness.

Medical complications of low calorie diets include electrolyte imbalance, cholelithiasis and gall bladder colics, elevations in liver enzymes, dehydration, constipation, hair loss and nutritional deficiencies.

Weight loss achieved through LCDs or VLCDs has not been shown to be better sustainable than more gradual weight loss achieved by other means. Indications for LCDs and VLCDs should be limited to patients who require rapid weight loss for medical reasons.

For those patients who do require a LCD or VLCD approach, most would benefit from continued partial meal replacements, medications or surgery to maintain weight loss after completing the program.

Given the medical risks inherent in a VLCD, it is important to ensure the integrity of the program to which you refer your patient. Do your own due diligence in exploring the various options in your area. Refer to Appendix A on page 89 for guidance on auditing commercial weight-loss programs for safety, ethics, and efficacy.

> ▸ **Pearl:** When energy intake falls below the level needed for energy balance, protein requirements increase by 1.75 g for every 100 kcal deficit. Without this increase in protein, there is a risk of disproportionate loss of lean muscle during the period of rapid weight loss.

PHYSICAL ACTIVITY

Patients and physicians tend to overestimate how much exercise contributes to weight loss — achieving even a modest negative energy balance through increased physical activity is a challenge. That said, the importance of exercise as a determinant of health cannot be overstated, and exercise does play a significant role in weight management.

> ▸ **Pearl:** Exercise lowers cardiovascular risk even if no weight is lost because it lowers blood pressure, reduces insulin resistance, improves lipid profile, enhances fibrinolysis, improves endothelial function, and enhances parasympathetic autonomic tone.

Exercise supports weight-management efforts by giving people a positive psychological boost. Exercise is uplifting and has been shown to be as effective as some SSRIs in the treatment of depression. Exercise is also health-promoting as it provides a regular reminder of the benefits of healthy living and can help people make healthy eating and behaviours habitual.

Exercise during weight loss and weight maintenance also helps minimize the loss of calorie-burning lean body mass, thereby preserving resting metabolic rate. Exercise also improves insulin sensitivity, resulting in lower insulin levels that may promote fat mobilization. New evidence also suggests that exercise may boost the size and number of the body's energy-burning mitochondria. Lastly, some "emotional" eaters may come to find emotional release from exercise and thereby find it easier to control emotionally triggered food intake.

One common hazard from overestimating the calories burned during exercise is that people reward their exercise with larger portions or high-calorie foods. It is useful to discuss calories burned through exercise to ward off this tendency. You can tell patients it would take a 15-minute fast-paced run to "exercise off" the calories in five small pieces of chocolate, a 30-minute walk to burn off one small cream-filled sponge cake, a half hour of jogging for one "sports drink," over two hours on a stationary bike to burn off 1.5 cups of high-calorie ice cream, and a seven-hour stroll to use up the calories in one typical fast-food meal.

> ▸ **Pearl:** Given that there are about 3,500 kcal in a pound of fat, "exercising off" that pound would require walking at a moderate pace for roughly 6–10 hours.

It is well documented that people who do not exercise during and following a weight management effort are far more likely to gain back the weight they have lost. Whether this is a function of the physiologic changes associated with exercise described above, or because of the psychological benefits of exercise, exercise appears to be an integral determinant of long-term success.

The exercise prescription you design will be dictated by what the particular patient is able to do and by what they actually enjoy doing. It is important to start at an exercise level that can be maintained without discouragement or injury. Patients with cardiovascular disease, diabetes, or other chronic disease should undergo a medical evaluation before initiating any exercise program more vigorous than walking. As fitness improves and weight loss occurs, increasing the intensity and duration of exercise will provide greater benefits.

The key is to match the physical activity prescription to the patient's abilities, needs and interests, with the ultimate clinical goal of achieving weight management and better health. A gradual moderate approach can enhance a patient's confidence and long-term adherence as they realize physical activity can be integrated into daily life. It is important to emphasize that exercise need not be gym-based or lengthy to be beneficial. From a weight-management perspective, multiple short bouts of exercise are just as, if not more, beneficial than longer single sessions. A study comparing groups randomized to either 10-minute exercise sessions or 30–40 minute sessions demonstrated that the short-bout exercisers actually logged more weekly minutes. Remind patients that whether they make one $30 deposit or three $10 deposits, at the end of the day they will have $30 in the account.

In the National Weight Control Registry where the average registrant lost 30 kg (67 lbs) and maintained that loss for more than five years, over 50% of registrants relied exclusively on walking for exercise. What this tells us is that the best exercise is something the patient can enjoy and sustain: walking, yard work, dancing, playing with children, or home improvement projects.

> ▸ **Pearl:** Have your patients aim for a minimum 150 minutes of exercise weekly and remind them that many brief exercise sessions are just as beneficial as fewer long ones. The total is what matters.

Patients also need to be taught that exercise need not be a structured, isolated, or physically demanding activity. Patients may consider using a pedometer to objectively quantify their daily activity levels. The pedometer can inspire minor changes to daily life, such as using a spot in the parking lot that is farthest from the door, taking the stairs instead of the elevator, or getting off the bus a stop or two early.

> ▸ **Pearl:** When using a pedometer, there is no "right" number of steps: 10,000 steps is only a reasonable goal for those who enjoy taking 10,000 steps. People who are miserable for the last 4,000 are likely to stop stepping altogether. The goal is "as many steps as you can enjoy."

BEHAVIOURAL INTERVENTIONS

The purpose of behaviour modification is to help patients identify and then modify the thought processes, eating and physical activity behaviours that contribute to their obesity.

There are a multitude of different behavioural approaches, and to date no single one has been shown to be better than another. There are three general principles in behaviour modification therapy. First, behavioural treatment should specify quantifiable goals (e.g., keeping a food diary or walking 10 minutes each day before breakfast). Specific goals make it easier to assess whether these have been attained, and if not, to initiate targeted problem solving.

> ▸ **Pearl:** Specific targets increase the likelihood of success. Setting a broad target of "exercising more" is much less likely to lead to a change in exercise pattern than setting a specific target of a daily 20-minute walk at a given time.

Second, behavioural therapy is process-oriented and helps patients develop realistic goals as well as a reasonable plan for reaching those goals. Planning and organization, rather than willpower and sacrifice, are considered keys to sustainable weight management.

Third, behavioural treatment prefers small over large changes. Setting small achievable goals allows patients to experience success, which can provide a solid foundation for additional lifestyle modifications. Drastic behavioural change is usually short-lived.

> ▸ **Pearl:** The single most important prerequisite for a successful behavioural intervention is the absence of hunger. Millions of years of evolutionary biology have taught our bodies how to find calories. Even the most intelligent and motivated patients will struggle with behavioural interventions if they are hungry. Only in the absence of hunger can a patient learn to practice thoughtful eating.

Behavioural therapy for obesity usually includes the following elements:
- Self-monitoring
- Stimulus control
- Social support
- Cognitive restructuring (thinking positively)
- Problem-solving skills
- Relapse intervention

Behavioural therapy can be provided in group or individual sessions and is often undertaken as a time-limited program. However, once an initial phase of weight reduction is completed, patients may still benefit from participating in weight maintenance programs.

Motivational Interviewing

Motivational interviewing (MI) is defined as "a client-centered, directive method for enhancing intrinsic motivation to change by exploring and resolving ambivalence." Motivational interviewing can be viewed as a patient-centered, therapist-directed personal exploration of the reasons for changing (in our case, to a healthier lifestyle).

MI involves an exploration of four main psychological elements:
1. Disadvantages of the status quo
2. Advantages of change
3. Optimism of change
4. Intention to change

While a thorough grounding in MI technique is far beyond the scope of this book, one of the most important points raised in descriptions of the method is the impact of counselling style on treatment outcomes. Confrontational counselling results in higher recidivism and worse outcomes. Conversely, reflective listening approaches increase patient response to treatment. Questions such as, "Why won't you change?" "How can you not be concerned about the medical risks of your weight?" and "Why can't you just do this?" will lead you and your patient nowhere.

Reflective listening involves reframing the above questions to promote discussion: "Does your weight cause you any medical or personal difficulties?" "What type of benefits do you see happening in your life if you do lose weight?" and "What types of beneficial changes do you think you can make this week?"

In this scenario, your patients not only present their own arguments for change, but also identify how they will achieve change and what outcomes they feel most confident and hopeful about reaching.

Cognitive Behavioural Therapy

Cognitive behavioural therapy (CBT) aims to modify thoughts, beliefs and assumptions that contribute to negative emotions or behaviours. There are many different modalities of CBT, including rational emotive therapy, interpersonal therapy, cognitive therapy, and cognitive analytic therapy, but for simplicity's sake we will use the term CBT to refer to any of these approaches. They share certain basic features, such as keeping a diary to record emotions, thoughts and/or behaviours, therapeutic questioning and testing of patient beliefs, gradual inclusion of activities that patients previously avoided, and trying out new ways of coping and reacting.

In the treatment of obesity, CBT aims to modify a patient's dysfunctional (from a weight perspective) eating behaviours, negative self-image, and perceived lack of self-control through the use of positive reframing and simple quantitative tools.

Constructive vs. Destructive Questions

Helping patients recognize the positive outcomes of their experiences is essential to foster behavioural change. Patients will often spend inordinate amounts of time contemplating what they perceive to be their failings, which is a pursuit that generates strong negative emotions. Eating foods they feel they ought not to, eating more than they had planned, or eating in a manner that they find upsetting can often plunge patients into a spiral of guilt where they dwell on questions such as "What's wrong with me?" or "Why can't I just do this?" The answers patients arrive at are often fraught with negativity: "You're a failure," "You're a quitter," or "This happens to you all the time." These answers do little to move a patient forward and may even be enough to make them give up.

Teaching patients to ask themselves more constructive, forward-looking questions and reframe their situation is helpful. Questions such as, "What can you do today that will help?" or "What can you do tomorrow to be proud of?" can refocus a patient's energies on the future, as can the explicit acceptance of human imperfection as a reality.

Forbidden Foods

One of the most common beliefs that needs to be reframed is the idea of "forbidden" foods. Every patient has their own particular food in mind here, but they are generally high in calories and low in nutritive value, and patients feel that they must be banished completely for the weight-loss effort to succeed. These are often a patient's comfort foods and inevitably something will occur that will lead the patient to indulge in them. The initial "transgression" may encourage a patient to consume a great deal of that particular food because they know they might not allow themselves that indulgence again. This can lead to a "write-off" day when many forbidden foods are consumed and the patient ends up feeling demoralized and guilty — just the thing to derail an entire weight-management effort.

There can be no forbidden foods in a sustainable weight-management program. Regardless of their calorie content or lack of nutritive value, all foods are allowed. If a patient feels that chocolate is their weakness, they must learn to consume the smallest amount of chocolate they need to be happy, rather than aim to consume no chocolate at all.

Food Diaries Revisited

The food diary can help identify both behavioural and organizational contributions to disordered eating. Patients can track the emotions associated with their meals and snacks and describe how particular meals and snacks make them feel. Identifying the emotions associated with foods enables patients and clinicians to begin to look for non-dietary behaviours or alternative dietary choices that might minimize both negative emotions and caloric intake.

The food diary can also be used to record the timing of meals, snacks and exercise as a way to understand behaviour and bring about change. A time log can help patients recognize the role hunger plays in disorganized eating. Common patterns that contribute to hunger and disorganized eating are:

- Not eating breakfast within 30 minutes of waking.
- Going longer than three hours between meals and snacks.
- Having fewer than 350 kcal in a meal or fewer than 150 kcal in a snack.
- Not including protein in all meals and snacks.
- Not fueling adequately for exercise lasting longer than 45 minutes (we recommend a 150-calorie carbohydrate-based snack either immediately preceding or during exercise).

Many patients are resistant to using food diaries because they see them as tools of judgment and negative reinforcement. You will need to explicitly reframe the use of the food diary and persuade patients that a food diary has three primary roles:

1. It provides caloric feedback to help with decision-making.
2. It helps identify patterns that may be compromising their efforts. Patients can be taught to track hunger, cravings and emotions to better answer questions like, "Why did I get hungry?"
3. It serves as a powerful tool in new habit cultivation. Every entry in the food diary reminds the patient of behaviours they are trying to change, and the more frequently they remind themselves of new possible behaviours, the more likely they are to incorporate these changes permanently.

> ▸ **Pearl:** While keeping a food diary may seem like a daunting task, patients can become quite proficient at it very quickly. Most people are creatures of habit and we tend to eat the same foods repeatedly, so as we learn the caloric content of our regular meals, keeping a food diary takes only as long as writing things down.

We have included a sample one-week food diary as an Appendix on page 92. Please feel free to photocopy it and distribute it to your patients.

Body Image

Body image dissatisfaction and body image distress can make weight-loss efforts more challenging. Dissatisfaction with body image can hinder a patient's efforts to exercise because they dread being seen in gym clothes. Unrealistic body image desires can cause patients who have lost medically significant amounts of weight to feel like failures. As noted earlier, body image dissatisfaction is also a major risk factor for disordered eating, which is often triggered by an episode of body image distress.

While a detailed treatment plan for body image disorder is beyond the scope of this book, you may want to recommend Dr. Thomas Cash's self-directed cognitive behavioural therapy workbook for body image, *The Body Image Workbook: An 8 step program for learning to like your looks* to patients in need of help. Dr. Cash is possibly the world's foremost expert on body image and he has validated the efficacy of the workbook in increasing body image satisfaction and decreasing body image distress in clinical trials. It is available from all major online book sellers and at many local libraries. The book's eight-stage program involves learning techniques for self-monitoring, relaxation, imaginal desensitization, rational response, and relapse prevention. "Workbook" is a very appropriate term for the title, as the book consists primarily of self-directed exercises, including over 40 self-discovery and change help sheets.

> ▸ **Pearl:** While it is unlikely that patients will model their body image desires on Barbie dolls, simply knowing that only one in 100,000 women share Barbie's proportions may help deal with body image perspective. It means that in all of Canada there are only about 30 real-life Barbies walking around, and they would be 5 feet 9 inches tall measuring 36-18-33.

As with everything in medicine, prevention is always preferable to treatment. There are a few strategies you can teach your patients to use to prevent them and possibly other family members from developing an unhealthy body image.

Advise your patients to:
- make their homes appearance-safe zones where family members are taught never to tease or bully each other about the way they look.
- not criticize their own appearance or clothes in front of their children, as this can cultivate unhealthy body images and unhealthy behaviours as children replicate parental behaviour.
- teach their children about media and commercials and the unrealistic messages they convey.
- not comment negatively on their children's choice of clothing, or more specifically, on how their clothing "makes them look."
- stop buying glossy diet, fitness, or fashion magazines.
- ask their children's school to consider adding classes on media awareness, and provide the school with the resource below.
- stop recommending or discouraging specific foods with messages tied to body image (eating that will make you/me fat, etc.). Shift the focus to health instead.

A fabulous resource for parents and schools for learning more about media and how to teach children to critically appraise advertising comes from the Canadian non-profit organization Media Awareness Network. You can find it on the Web at www.media-awareness.ca. You will find lesson plans and resources for parents and schools along with online games for children.

[CHAPTER 9: MEDICATION]

The U.S. National Institutes of Health recommends that pharmacotherapy for obesity be prescribed only in conjunction with a planned weight-management program. Even as part of a program, the efficacy of existing medications is modest at best, with weight losses of 5%–10% in patients with moderate obesity. Given that obesity is a chronic condition and that pharmacotherapy is a treatment rather than a cure, discontinuation of pharmacotherapy is generally associated with weight regain. Most patients must therefore continue on these medications indefinitely. Pharmacotherapy for the treatment of obesity is comparable to lifelong pharmacologic treatment for other chronic conditions such as hypertension, diabetes, or hypercholesterolemia.

Pharmacotherapy can help patients lower their body's caloric intake either by decreasing caloric absorption or decreasing dietary intake. For example, if an appetite suppressant allows a patient to be satisfied with 500 fewer calories a day, they will initially lose weight at a rate of roughly 0.45 kg (1 lb) per week. This rate of weight loss will slow as the number of calories their shrinking body burns decreases. Eventually a new homeostasis will be reached, where the calories they ingest are equal to their total daily energy expenditure, and weight loss will cease. Medication may also be useful in helping a patient whose lifestyle effort has proven to be non-sustainable (due to an overly restrictive diet or a constant battle with hunger). Adding pharmacotherapy may turn a regimen that produces suffering into one that is manageable or even effortless.

Patients who are unable to achieve a sustainable healthy body weight on their own despite a strong desire for weight loss, but who are unwilling to accept the idea of long-term pharmacotherapy, should not be started on medication. The patient's reluctance to consider the possibility of lifelong need reflects their lack of acceptance that obesity is a chronic lifelong disease.

Unfortunately, the troubled history of obesity drugs such as amphetamines, phen-fen and other sympathomimetic agents has resulted in skepticism regarding the role of anti-obesity agents. Given the well-defined and predictable side effect profiles of current agents (orlistat, sibutramine), it would seem that these drugs should be prescribed with the same caution you might use to prescribe other medications, but not more.

The hesitation of health care professionals and regulators to fully endorse anti-obesity medications may reflect their misconception that obesity is largely a personal choice rather than a chronic illness — that these patients do not "deserve" long-term medications to help them manage their weight.

To date, we know that:

- combining anti-obesity drugs and lifestyle modification is superior to lifestyle modification alone in achieving and maintaining a target weight loss of 5%–10%.
- discontinuation of anti-obesity medication generally results in weight regain and medication should therefore be continued as long as there is continued benefit. Benefit includes weight maintenance as well as weight loss. Long-term studies are only available for sibutramine and orlistat.
- despite demonstrated improvements in risk factors, co-morbidities, and quality of life, we are still years away from being able to demonstrate the impact of anti-obesity medications on overall mortality.
- there is no evidence that current anti-obesity medications are associated with pulmonary hypertension, valvular dysfunction, or other cardiovascular abnormalities associated with earlier obesity medications.
- there are no obesity medications currently in use that produce physiologic dependence or addiction.

Amazingly, despite the fact that obesity is the second-most preventable cause of death in North America, there are still only four drugs approved for its management.

SIBUTRAMINE

Sibutramine is a satiogenic drug that acts by inhibiting serotonin and norepinephrine intake, thereby amplifying the natural feeling of satiety following a meal. It may also have modest thermogenic effects on energy metabolism. It is generally prescribed at a dose of 10–15 mg once daily.

The key utility of this drug in the long-term management of obesity is to enhance satiety and thereby decrease caloric intake. Properly used, it enables most patients to reduce portion size and restrict overeating. As sibutramine is not formally an appetite suppressant, patients should continue regular intake of satiating foods (i.e., low energy density, high-fibre, low-GI, high-protein foods). Sibutramine seems to work by amplifying the body's natural satiety signal. Since this usually takes 20 to 40 minutes to develop, "slow" foods can enhance drug efficacy, as can eating low-energy density foods, such as salads, before a meal. It is also important to note that sibutramine does not help patients reduce the intake of liquid calories (soft drinks, alcohol) as these do not elicit a natural satiety response.

Sibutramine is generally well tolerated. Common side effects are similar to those seen with other serotonin-norepinephrine reuptake inhibitors (SNRIs) and include xerostomia, insomnia, hyperhidrosis, and constipation. Sibutramine also consistently leads to an increase in heart rate of 4–5 beats/minute and in some instances it can provoke palpitations. The increase in heart rate can be prevented or reversed with exercise training.

Sibutramine's effect on blood pressure is more complex and variable. While sibutramine may lead to a modest increase (1–2 mmHg) in individuals with normal blood pressure, there is now evidence to suggest that sibutramine may in fact lower blood pressure in hypertensive individuals. This effect is likely due to the recently described central sympatholytic "clonidine-like" effect of sibutramine that results in reduced peripheral sympathetic activity. Recent studies also demonstrate sibutramine's positive effects on sleep apnea, endothelial dysfunction, and left-ventricular hypertrophy. Sibutramine-induced weight loss is likely to further reduce blood pressure levels.

> ▸ **Pearl:** Sibutramine is not contraindicated in hypertensive patients with well-controlled blood pressure.

Recent findings suggest that sibutramine can increase the risk for non-fatal myocardial infarction and other cardiovascular complications in high-risk patients. This finding has led to the withdrawal of sibutramine in many European countries.

As with other SNRIs, combining sibutramine with other centrally active drugs should be done cautiously. While the co-administration of sibutramine with SSRIs or other SNRIs is contraindicated in some countries, in others (e.g., the U. S.) prescription information only warns clinicians to carefully monitor patients for the serotonin syndrome, which is a rare and potentially fatal condition (see Table 8 below). Sibutramine is absolutely contraindicated in patients on monoamine oxidase inhibitors (MAO).

Serotonin syndrome encompasses a wide constellation of symptoms commonly subdivided into mental, autonomic, and somatic symptoms. These are summarized below:

Table 8: Revised diagnostic criteria for serotonin syndrome

1. Addition of a serotonergic agent to an already established treatment (or increase in dosage) and manifestation of at least four major symptoms or three major symptoms plus two minor ones.

Mental (cognitive and behavioural) symptoms
Major symptoms: confusion, elevated mood, coma, or semicoma
Minor symptoms: agitation and nervousness, insomnia

Autonomic symptoms
Major symptoms: fever, hyperhidrosis
Minor symptoms: tachycardia, tachypnea and dyspnea, diarrhea, low or high blood pressure

Neurological symptoms
Major symptoms: myoclonus, tremors, chills, rigidity, hyperreflexia
Minor symptoms: impaired coordination, mydriasis, akathisia

2. These symptoms must not correspond to a psychiatric disorder, or its aggravation, which occurred before the patient took the serotonergic agent.
3. Infectious, metabolic, endocrine, or toxic causes must be excluded.
4. A neuroleptic treatment must not have been introduced, nor its dose increased, before the symptoms appeared.

Source: **Birmes, P. et al.** Serotonin syndrome: a brief review. *Canadian Medical Association Journal* 168; 2003.

ORLISTAT

Orlistat is a gastrointestinal lipase inhibitor that reduces intestinal absorption of dietary fat by as much as 30%. It is generally prescribed at a dose of 120 mg tid (with each meal), although a lower-dose version is now available over the counter in some countries. If patients consume too much fat (>~60 grams a day), they will experience severe and urgent side effects (see below). For patients whose diets are low in fat, orlistat will likely not have much effect: without the calories from fat to malabsorb, the drug will not induce a caloric deficit. As gastrointestinal lipase is produced during each meal, orlistat must be taken before every fat-containing meal. This drug is best prescribed for patients whose daily caloric intake includes a significant amount of fat.

> ▸ **Pearl:** Orlistat has no effect on calories from carbohydrates, protein or alcohol.

Several clinical studies document the efficacy of orlistat in reducing body weight, with resulting improvements in waist circumference, glycemic control, and dyslipidemia. Effects on lipid levels may be partially independent of weight loss. In some countries, orlistat is specifically approved for use in patients with type 2 diabetes.

Due to its mode of action, the primary side effects of orlistat are gastrointestinal. These include bloating, flatulence, oily discharge, spotting, and urgent diarrhea. Dietary inconsistencies result in unpredictable side effects and "accidents" that can lead to embarrassing situations. It may therefore be a good idea to start treatment on week-ends only, and to perhaps discourage its use in patients for whom bathroom breaks are challenging during a typical day (long daily commutes or jobs where they do not have ready access to bathroom facilities).

Regular use of orlistat may affect levels of fat-soluble vitamins. As many patients start out with deficiencies in Vitamin D, prescribing a regular supplement to be taken between meals may be advisable. Orlistat may also interfere with vitamin K absorption, so patients on warfarin will need closer monitoring of international normalized ratio (INR).

Orlistat also interferes with the bioavailability of lipophilic drugs. This has been described particularly for cyclosporine A, for which orlistat markedly reduces intestinal absorption.

Table 9: Comparison of anti-obesity drugs orlistat and sibutramine

Feature	Orlistat	Sibutramine
Drug class	Gastric and pancreatic lipase inhibitor	Noradrenaline (norepinephrine) and serotonin reuptake inhibitor (via active metabolites M1 and M2)
Mechanism of action	Prevents absorption of ≈30% of dietary intake.	Enhances satiety (decreases food intake)
Target population	Initial BMI of >30 kg/m², or >27kg/m² (US) or >28 kg/m² (UK) with risk factors[a]	Initial BMI of >30 kg/m², or >27 kg/m² with risk factors[a]
Usual dosage[b]	120 mg orally three times daily with each main meal	10-15 mg orally once daily with or without food
Special instructions	Patients must take a multivitamin supplement (2 hours before a dose). No dose should be taken if a meal is missed or contains no fat.	Blood pressure monitoring is required before and during therapy.
Contraindications	Chronic malabsorption syndrome, cholestasis, pregnant/ nursing women, hypersensitivity to the drug	Coronary artery disease, congestive heart failure, arrhythmias, stroke, severe renal or hepatic impairment, poorly controlled or uncontrolled hypertension, anorexia nervosa, patients taking monoamine oxidase inhibitors[c] or other serotonergic drugs
Use with caution	History of hyperoxaluria or calcium oxalate nephrolithiasis	History of hypertension, seizures, narrow angle glaucoma
Use in children	UK: Not recommended US: Safety and efficacy have not been established	UK: Drug not available US: Safety and efficacy in pediatric patients (>16 years of age) have not been established.
Abuse potential	As with any weight-loss agent, the potential exists for misuse in inappropriate patient populations (e.g., with anorexia nervosa or bulimia).	Physicians should evaluate patients for history of abuse and observe closely for signs of misuse or abuse
Adverse effects:		
Most common	Gastrointestinal (oily spotting or stool, flatus, increased fecal urgency)	Headache, dry mouth, anorexia, insomnia, constipation
Cardiovascular	None	Increased blood pressure and heart rate
Potential drug interactions	Decreased absorption of fat-soluble vitamins	May potentiate action of monoamine oxidase inhibitors (see contraindications) and drugs that increase blood pressure or heart rate; metabolism may be inhibited by Cytochrome P4503A1 inhibitors.

[a] Hypertension, diabetes mellitus, dyslipidemia

[b] Taken in conjunction with a reduced-calorie diet. In patients taking orlistat the diet should contain ≈30% of calories from fat

[c] Or within two weeks of monoamine oxidase inhibitors therapy

Source: Better than slim chances for orlistat and sibutramine to promote weight loss. *Drugs & Therapy Perspectives*, 15, 12; 1-6: 2000.

Phentermine and Diethylpropion

These sympathicomimetic drugs are only approved for short-term treatment of obesity (up to 12 weeks), though in the U.S. they are often used in pulse therapy for years at a time (12 weeks on, four weeks off). They act by inhibiting the reuptake of norepinephrine into nerve terminals, thus increasing the activity of the sympathetic nervous system. Side effects can include dysrhythmias, hypertension, chest pain, and insomnia. Traditionally these drugs were thought to have the potential for abuse, but we are not aware of any documented cases of addiction. If they had addictive properties, we would expect tolerance to develop, yet studies on both medications demonstrate no loss of efficacy or need for increased dosing to maintain weight loss.

Contraindications to phentermine or diethylpropion include advanced or symptomatic coronary artery disease, uncontrolled hypertension, hyperthyroid states, glaucoma, concurrent tricyclic antidepressant use, and administration of an MAO inhibitor within 14 days.

OFF-LABEL AND EMERGING PHARMACOLOGIC OBESITY THERAPIES

Topiramate/Zonisamide

Topiramate is approved for use as an antiepileptic drug and for the treatment of migraines. After weight loss was reported as a common side effect in topiramate-treated seizure disorder patients, trials were initiated and are currently underway to evaluate its efficacy as a formal weight-loss medication. In clinical seizure disorder trials it was associated with weight loss that continued beyond one year. Topiramate also seems to reduce binge-eating frequency in patients with binge-eating disorder.

Side effects of topiramate, especially at high doses, can be quite severe and include paresthesias, somnolence, and difficulty concentrating. It has also been associated with metabolic acidosis.

In our experience, topiramate at doses as low as 50–75 mg a day can be helpful in augmenting weight loss and/or reducing binge eating. However, if it is not effective at these doses, it should not be increased.

Zonisamide is an antiepileptic drug that has serotonergic and dopaminergic activity. It has also been associated with weight loss and is being studied for the treatment of obesity and binge-eating disorders. It is associated with fewer central nervous system side effects than topiramate.

Metformin

Treatment with metformin is associated with a 2.5% loss of body weight. Although it does not produce the 5% weight loss required to be considered a "weight-loss drug," it can be very useful in overweight individuals at high risk for diabetes.

In the United Kingdom Prospective Diabetes Study (UKPDS) of diet-treated overweight patients with type 2 diabetes, the addition of metformin reduced the risk for diabetes-related end points, diabetes-related deaths, and all causes of mortality. Obese patients with type 2 diabetes should be considered good candidates for metformin therapy even if their diabetic control through lifestyle intervention is adequate according to laboratory criteria. As noted earlier, metformin can be prescribed alongside antipsychotic medications to help attenuate iatrogenic weight gain. It is also considered first-line therapy in the treatment of PCOS.

Side effects of metformin can include gastrointestinal disturbances and rarely, hyperchloremic metabolic acidosis. Metformin should be used cautiously in patients with renal insufficiency.

> ▸ **Pearl:** Patients exhibiting insulin resistance and hyperinsulinemia may benefit from metformin as this drug's mechanism of action can reduce hyperinsulinemia and potentially improve the metabolic parameters affected by insulin.

Acarbose and Miglitol
Acarbose and miglitol are competitive inhibitors of pancreatic amylase and/or intestinal alpha glycosidases, which produce a delay of intestinal glucose absorption and reduce the availability of glucose for energy use. This in turn reduces postprandial insulin and glucose peaks. Side effects of acarbose and miglitol are mainly gastrointestinal, including bloating, abdominal pain, and diarrhea.

In theory, these agents might reduce total energy intake by modifying glucose availability or oral glucose intake secondary to gastrointestinal side effects; however, they are currently not recommended nor approved for the management of obesity.

Pramlintide
Pramlintide is a synthetic analog of human amylin (a peptide hormone secreted by pancreatic beta cells along with insulin in response to nutrient stimuli) that slows gastric emptying, reduces postprandial rises in blood glucose concentrations, and improves $HbA1_c$ concentrations in diabetic patients. Unlike insulin and many anti-diabetic medications, pramlintide is associated with modest weight loss and is currently under study as a weight-loss aid.

In 2006, a phase II study reported that after 16 weeks of therapy, subjects taking pramlintide had lost an average of 3.8–6 kg (8.3–13.4 lbs). Pramlinitide is currently undergoing investigation in combination with a long-acting leptin analogue metreleptin for obesity treatment.

GLP-1 Agonists
GLP-1 agonists (e.g. exenatide, liraglutide) are long-acting synthetic peptides that act as GLP-1 agonists and are used as adjunctive therapy for patients with type 2 diabetes. Their use is associated with dose-dependant weight loss in patients with type 2 diabetes who are not well controlled on oral agents.

Bupropion
Bupropion is approved for the treatment of depression and for smoking cessation. It is also useful in the prevention of smoking-cessation-associated weight gain. Treatment

with bupropion is associated with significant weight loss at six months compared with placebo, and this has been shown to be largely maintained during a six-month treatment arm extension. Weight loss achieved with bupropion results primarily from the loss of fat mass.

Side effects include dry mouth, agitation, constipation, and insomnia. It is contraindicated in patients with a history of seizure disorders because it may trigger seizures in a dose-dependent fashion. It is also ill-advised to prescribe bupropion to a patient with any significant anxiety disorder as it is liable to exacerbate that condition.

When indicated in obese patients with depression, bupropion may help promote weight loss without producing significant side effects or worsening cardiovascular risk. It can therefore can be considered first-line therapy for depression in obese patients without contraindications.

Bupropion is also currently being assessed as an adjuvant treatment for binge-eating disorder. It may work to diminish food cravings just as it diminishes nicotine cravings.

Selective Serotonin Reuptake Inhibitors
SSRIs, which are approved for the treatment of depression, may help facilitate weight loss in the short run. Treatment with fluoxetine at a dose of 60 mg/day (three times the usual dose for the treatment of depression) was associated with weight loss at six months and one year of 4.8 kg and 2.4 kg (10.6 lbs and 5.3 lbs), respectively. These results were short-lived, however. Continued use of the drug for more than six months was associated with weight gain, suggesting that the drug has limited usefulness as a short-term anti-obesity treatment. Similar results have been seen with other SSRIs.

For obese patients with depression who have contraindications to treatment with bupropion, SSRIs may be preferred over other antidepressants, many of which cause weight gain (including MAOIs, TCAs, SNRIs, antipsychotics, and mirtazapine).

Fluoxetine (60 mg/day) has been approved in the treatment of binge-eating disorder. Side effects may include sexual dysfunction, somnolence, insomnia, agitation, diarrhea, and tremor.

Human Recombinant Growth Hormone
Human recombinant growth hormone (HrGH) promotes loss of fat mass while increasing lean body mass in GH-deficient children and adults. However, when used in obese patients, HrGH has not been shown to be an effective weight-loss aid. Its use also increases insulin resistance. A synthetic fragment of HrGH is currently being studied for obesity treatment, but it is still in early clinical trials.

Testosterone
Testosterone and the anabolic steroid, oxandrolone, have been reported to reduce visceral fat. While testosterone is indicated in the treatment of hypogonadal men, it has yet to have proven utility in the treatment of obesity.

Methylphenidate

Widely used as treatment for ADHD, this compound may have a specific role in obese patients with this condition. The issue of additional anorexic effects is being explored. Methylphenidate's mechanism of action as a dopamine and norepinephrine reuptake inhibitor may affect appetite by increasing synaptic dopamine and, in so doing, decrease the dopamine-mediated reinforcing comfort of food.

In a study looking at the effect of a single dose of methylphenidate before the consumption of a highly palatable meal (pizza) by obese men, those who were given 5 mg of methylphenidate prior to the meal consumed 34% fewer calories than those who were given placebo.

OVER-THE-COUNTER SUPPLEMENTS

Over-the-counter dietary supplements are widely used by people attempting to lose weight, but evidence to support their efficacy and safety is limited. Despite the lack of proven value, and an embarrassing lack of governmental regulations governing such products, a large industry promotes their use.

A number of herbal and plant preparations are marketed to treat obesity, but there are few controlled trials to document their efficacy. A major problem with herbal preparations is that they are not pure, and may contain substances other than the active ingredient that are not necessarily safe. Health Canada has been kept busy recalling nutraceutical weight-loss aids due to the inclusion of prescription weight-loss medication in formulations (usually sibutramine or phentermine).

Commonly included ingredients in these natural weight-loss preparations are some combination of: chitosan, chromium picolinate, conjugated linoleic acid (CLA), dehydroepiandrosterone (DHEA), ephedra sinica, guar gum, garcinia cambogia, glucomannan, guarana, hoodia, hydroxy-methylbutyrate, plantago psyllium, pyruvate, and yohimbine. These compounds have not yet been shown to be effective in the treatment of obesity, and without publication of clinical trials, safety and drug interaction data is not available. Of the products for which data are available, efficacy and safety data are far from impressive:

Ephedrine (a synthetic adrenergic drug) and related compounds (ephedra alkaloids) has been shown to have both anorectic and thermogenic properties. These properties were enhanced by co-administration with caffeine, a xanthine compound that potentiates the effects of ephedrine by preventing the breakdown of norepinephrine in the synaptic junction. Due to the association of ephedrine and related compounds with severe cardiovascular events, the FDA banned ephedra from use in dietary supplements for obesity.

Olestra is a non-caloric fat substitute consisting of sucrose esterified with fatty acids. It does not undergo lipolysis, nor is it absorbed. Its principal side effects are mild to moderate gastrointestinal symptoms. There is no evidence that olestra consumption changes total energy intake, but it is associated with a reduction in energy consumed as fat in people whose fat intake is moderate to heavy.

DHEA and **CLA** were shown to affect weight loss in animal studies, but to date human studies have been negative. Therefore, there seems to be no place for these agents in the treatment of obesity.

PGX (PolyGlycopleX) is a non-starch polysaccharide (fibre) that has a high water-absorbing capacity and is thus sold as a satiety promoting supplement. Clinical trials on its use as a weight-loss agent are underway.

Orlistat has recently been approved in the U.S. in a half-strength over-the-counter dose.

▸ **Pearl:** If a patient is convinced that "natural" is synonymous with "safe," you may consider pointing out that tobacco is quite natural, as are many mushrooms that could land them in hospital.

[CHAPTER 10: SURGERY]

The term bariatric surgery refers to gastrointestinal surgical interventions conducted to produce sustainable weight loss. At present, bariatric surgery is the only therapeutic modality that can truly claim to produce sustainable weight loss, halt or resolve co-morbidities, and substantially reduce mortality in patients with morbid obesity. Reduction in mortality is largely attributable to a reduced risk of dying from complications of diabetes, cardiovascular disease, and cancer.

The advent of the laparoscopic approach to bariatric surgery has significantly reduced morbidity and mortality, and has promoted rapid recovery from surgery. Best outcomes are achieved by interdisciplinary teams working in high-volume centres, and results are largely dependent on appropriate patient selection and follow-up. Successful weight loss after bariatric surgery is generally defined as at least 50% of excess body weight lost (EBWL) or 20%–35% of initial body weight.

> ▸ **Pearl:** The American Society for Metabolic and Bariatric Surgery (ASMBS) has an established accreditation procedure that indicates excellence in bariatric surgery based on safe bariatric surgical care with excellent short- and long-term outcomes. The designation, Bariatric Surgery Center of Excellence, is accorded to centres that meet the ASMBS criteria.

The generally accepted indication for gastrointestinal surgery for weight loss is BMI >40 or BMI >35 complicated by weight-related co-morbidities. The clinician should view these weight parameters as a guide rather than a rule, as patients with multiple or severe weight-related co-morbidities and BMI <35 may also be considered for surgery.

The three classes of surgical procedures most commonly used to produce weight loss are:

1. **Gastric restriction** (adjustable gastric banding)

2. **Combined gastric restriction and malabsorption** (Roux-en-Y gastric bypass)

3. **Malabsorption** (biliopancreatic diversion)

The mean percentage excess body weight loss for all procedures is approximately 60%. In addition to the weight loss, a substantial majority of patients with diabetes, hyperlipidemia, hypertension, and/or obstructive sleep apnea who undergo surgery experience complete resolution or improvement of these co-morbid conditions.

The operative mortality (mortality at 30 days or less) is reported to be 0.1% for the purely restrictive procedures, 0.5% for gastric bypass, and 1.1% for biliopancreatic diversion.

Non-fatal complications vary with the type of surgery. The most frequent are:
- dumping syndrome, consisting of rapid gastric emptying, abdominal cramps, and nausea (0.3% for restrictive and 14.6% for combination surgeries).
- vitamin/mineral deficiency, most commonly involving B12, iron, calcium, folate and fat soluble vitamins (1.6% for restrictive and 11% for combination surgeries).
- vomiting/nausea (8.5% for restrictive and 2.6% for combination surgeries).
- staple line failure (1.5% for restrictive and 6% for combination surgeries).
- infection (3.1% for restrictive and 5.3% for combination surgeries).
- stenosis/bowel obstruction (2.2% for restrictive and 2.7% for combination surgeries).
- ulceration (1.2% for both restrictive and combination surgeries).
- bleeding (0.5% for restrictive and 0.9% for combination surgeries).
- splenic injury (0.2% for restrictive and 8% for combination surgeries).

Source: **Abell TL et al.** Gastrointestinal complications of bariatric surgery: Diagnosis and Therapy. *Am J Med Sci.* 331 (4): 214-218 (2006).

While post-operative bariatric surgical patients also have a much higher risk of gallstones, this is due to weight loss following surgery and not to the surgery itself.

▶ **Pearl:** Gallstone formation may be inhibited by the post-operative use of ursodeoxycholic acid 500 mg bid until the cessation of rapid weight loss. This approach may also be used with any weight-management strategy resulting in rapid (>1.4 kg or 3 lbs/week) weight loss.

Bacterial overgrowth and diarrhea can also be indirect consequences of bariatric surgery.

For the vast majority of patients who meet surgical selection criteria, the benefits of weight loss will greatly outweigh the risks of surgery, including possible complications, pain, and anxiety. Even when the inconveniences of dietary restrictions are taken into account, quality of life almost invariably improves for these patients after surgery. Improvements arise from the achievement of weight loss, relief from debilitating and potentially fatal co-morbid conditions, and improved social and economic opportunities. To counsel patients effectively, you should have a basic understanding of the various bariatric surgical options. Here is a brief description of the most common procedures:

ADJUSTABLE GASTRIC BANDING

This procedure involves creating a small upper gastric pouch (15 mL–45 mL in volume) by placing a band around the upper aspects of the stomach into which the esophagus empties. For this operation to be successful, the outlet of the pouch must be quite small (10 mm in diameter).

The primary aim of gastric banding is to create a mechanical restriction that limits the passage of food from the distal esophagus and small gastric pouch to the digestive tract. However, the operation's success comes not from the mechanical obstruction itself, but from the reduction in food intake, as patients experience earlier satiety when their newly small gastric pouch is filled. This enables patients to severely restrict portion sizes without feeling undue hunger.

Purely restrictive operations, especially gastric banding, may boast lower surgical risk than combination surgeries, but their effectiveness is not always dependable, in part because it is possible to "beat" the surgery by consuming high-calorie liquids (cream, milkshakes, etc.) which can still pass easily into the digestive tract.

Because of the procedure's simplicity, the adjustable gastric band is replacing vertical banded gastroplasty as the restrictive procedure of choice. The tension of the band and hence the size of the outlet is adjustable post-operatively by injecting or removing saline from a percutaneous silicone access port. Very recently, a wireless, telemetric adjustment system has been developed to permit non-invasive adjustments.

The band generally requires periodic adjustments, and it is important to ensure that a patient considering this procedure lives near a centre or clinic where adjustments can be made. Adjustable gastric banding also carries the risk of port infections, slippage, erosion, and other mechanical complications, including rare occurrences of complete outlet obstruction. While in theory adjustable gastric bands are easily removable, this generally results in rapid weight regain.

While purely restrictive procedures do not directly lead to deficiencies attributable to malabsorption, stomal stenoses resulting in markedly reduced food intake can lead to severe caloric, protein, and other nutritional deficits.

ROUX-EN-Y GASTRIC BYPASS

This procedure combines gastric restriction with intestinal bypass and is currently the most commonly performed surgical intervention worldwide for obesity treatment.

In a Roux-en-Y gastric bypass, the cardia is separated from the remainder of the stomach, creating a small gastric reservoir measuring approximately 10 mL. This reservoir is then anastomosed to a segment of the proximal jejunum, while the balance of the stomach and the jejunum proximal to the anastomosis are left in place as a blind limb.

Roux-en-Y gastric bypass affects weight through several mechanisms. The small gastric reservoir restricts intake, while the bypassed jejunal segment causes a degree of malabsorption and often leads to dumping syndrome in response to high-sugar liquid meals, thereby attenuating patients' sugar consumption. In addition, novel findings point to a specific effect of bypassing the duodenum and proximal ileum on glucose metabolism leading to notable improvement in glycemic control.

Roux-en-Y bypass procedures are associated with micronutrient (mineral and vitamin) and macronutrient (protein and calorie) deficiencies to a greater extent than purely restrictive procedures, but to a lesser extent than biliopancreatic diversion.

Roux-en-Y bypass surgery can lead to metabolic and nutritional complications, and patients should be monitored regularly following surgery. Patients are vulnerable to the development of iron deficiency anemia (especially in menstruating women) and vitamin B12 and folate deficiencies. Vitamin D and calcium deficiencies are less frequent than with biliopancreatic diversion and protein malnutrition is rare. To prevent deficiencies, oral multivitamin preparations containing iron, folate, B12, and vitamin D should be given to patients undergoing this bariatric surgery. Women should be placed on a calcium supplement.

Weight loss following Roux-en-Y gastric bypass surgery peaks at 65%–80% of excess body weight 12 to 18 months after surgery, and at five years mean excess weight loss ranges from 50%–60%, or about a 25% loss of total pre-surgical weight.

BILIOPANCREATIC DIVERSION (BPD) AND DUODENAL SWITCH

This procedure combines gastric restriction with intestinal malabsorption. In a BPD, a subtotal gastrectomy is performed, leaving a gastric pouch 200 mL–500 mL in volume. The distal 250 cm of the small intestine is divided into proximal and distal segments. The distal segment is anastomosed to the gastric remnant and the proximal segment is anastomosed to the distal ileum 50 cm from the ileocecal valve.

BPD also maintains weight loss through restriction and malabsorption. Malabsorption is much more marked than with a Roux-en-Y gastric bypass, as digestion and absorption bypasses virtually the entire small intestine, except for the 50 cm ileal segment.

Consequently, patients undergoing BPD are prone to more serious and troublesome metabolic complications, including protein malnutrition, iron, folate, B12, and lipid-soluble vitamin deficiencies. Patients should be encouraged to consume ample protein, and to take iron, folic acid, calcium, vitamin D, vitamin A, and vitamin B12 supplements. Vitamin K should also be supplemented if INR is found to be above 1.4. Due to its much higher risk of surgical morbidity, this procedure is commonly reserved for patients with super-morbid obesity.

A variant of this procedure is BPD with duodenal switch. This involves a partial sleeve gastrectomy, preserving the pylorus, as well as the creation of a Roux limb with a short common channel. It differs from BPD in terms of the portion of the stomach removed, and because it preserves the pylorus.

Its use is also advocated for patients with super-morbid obesity (BMI >50) and it may entail slightly fewer metabolic complications.

At present, both surgeries are considered viable first-line surgical treatments for patients with super-morbid obesity.

EXPERIMENTAL AND LESS-ESTABLISHED PROCEDURES

Vertical Sleeve Gastrectomy

Vertical sleeve gastrectomy (VSG) is a new technique indicated for patients with super-morbid obesity as an initial stage of surgical management. The procedure consists of a laparoscopic partial gastrectomy, in which most of the greater curvature of the stomach is removed and a tubular stomach is created, which is small in capacity and resistant to stretching due to the absence of the fundus. The procedure itself may be described as purely restrictive, but the removal of the stomach brings about hormonal changes that promote weight loss. The removal of 85% of the patient's stomach virtually eliminates ghrelin production. Given ghrelin's role in hunger, the absence of the hormone means that patients do not feel hunger and have an easier time consuming small portions and making fewer calorie-dense food choices. We do not yet know whether ghrelin production increases over time, but some patients have described a gradual return of cravings and hunger.

With VSG, patients experience an average 33% loss of excess weight in one year. For patients with super-morbid obesity, this weight loss is enough to decrease the risk of the more technically rigorous laparoscopic Roux-en-Y gastric bypass. Its relative technical ease also makes VSG possible as an isolated bariatric procedure for high-risk surgical patients.

Intragastric Balloon Placement
The intragastric balloon is a temporary option for weight loss in moderately obese patients. Using endoscopic surgery, a soft saline-filled balloon is placed into the patient's stomach. We assume that the distension of the balloon promotes satiety, while its physical size provides some physical restriction.

With intragastric balloon placement, mean excess body weight loss is reported to be around 40%–45%, however recent studies indicate that only 26% of the patients maintain 90% or more of that weight loss over one year.

As with the VSG, intragastric balloon placement is technically quite easy when compared with the Roux-en-Y gastric bypass. It can also be used to produce preoperative weight loss in super morbidly obese patients before they undergo more definitive bariatric procedures.

Implantable Gastric Stimulator
Originally designed for the treatment of gastroparesis, implantable gastric stimulators (IGSs) have recently attracted interest as a means of augmenting sustainable weight loss. Clinical trials investigating different variations of these devices are currently underway.

VBLOC Therapy
Consideration of VBLOC therapy as a weight-management strategy arose after appetite and weight reductions were noted in patients who had undergone vagotomies. VBLOC involves a surgically implanted device that delivers high-frequency, low-energy electrical signals to block vagal nerve transmission. It is thought that weight loss is mediated by the interruption of hunger signals that travel via the vagus nerve to the brain, though the exact mechanism of action has yet to be elucidated. VBLOC therapy is currently in the clinical trial stage.

PREOPERATIVE PATIENT SELECTION AND PREPARATION

Before patients undergo bariatric surgery, it is very important to address their expectations. Preoperative and post-operative education must aim to confront the common patient belief that post-surgical weight loss will be effortless and that they will achieve their "dream" weight.

Patients need to understand that surgical procedures are unlikely to return them to an "ideal" weight as defined by BMI, and that the primary goal is to reduce the risks of morbidity and mortality associated with their pre-surgical weight. You must also clearly spell out the potential adverse effects from these procedures and be sure patients understand the dietary and behavioural changes that go hand in hand with surgery.

> ▶ **Pearl:** Many patients feel tremendous guilt even contemplating surgery. They feel they are choosing the easy way out and that this marks them as failures. Explain to these patients that undergoing bariatric surgery is a very significant commitment that also requires dramatic lifestyle changes. In choosing to undergo surgery they are accepting far more risk and require as much if not more courage than those who are trying to manage their weight without surgery.

Psychological Impact of Surgery

The psychological stability of surgical candidates should be evaluated to assess their willingness and ability to adjust to the changes mandated by the surgery. Some patients consciously or unconsciously use their weight as a means to withdraw from social interaction or push away intimacy. For some patients, the inevitable weight loss associated with bariatric surgery can be quite distressing and rates of suicide in post-bariatric surgery patients are in fact higher than among weight-matched controls.

Mental health and psychosocial status, including social relations and employment opportunities, improve for the majority of people after bariatric surgery, contributing to improved quality of life. Obesity surgery also has a positive effect on affective and anxiety disorders.

Although most studies show optimistic results and report broad psychosocial improvement, a minority of patients do not benefit psychologically from surgery. Between 5%–10% of bariatric surgery patients divorce or separate following surgery. Partnerships in which there was considerable conflict before the operation are probably least likely to cope with the stress of the new situation.

Recurrence of addictive behaviours has been noted, including gambling, alcohol, and drug use. Patients with a history of addiction need to be carefully counseled and monitored after surgery.

These and similar problems are best addressed by involving mental health experts from the initial pre-surgical evaluation. Continued counselling and support groups are often helpful following the surgery.

> ▶ **Pearl:** The pre-surgical psychological evaluation should be performed by a psychiatrist or clinical psychologist with special interest in this population. If this expertise is lacking, you should seek out a new surgical centre for your patients.

POST-OPERATIVE PLASTIC SURGERY

While massive weight loss brings improvements in health status and quality of life, physical sequelae due to symptomatic skin redundancy will require further treatment. Areas affected include the arms, breasts, abdomen, back, and thighs. Patients who have undergone open rather than laparoscopic procedures often face the risk of incisional hernias due to poor support from incised abdominal musculature.

Cosmetic procedures include abdominal panniculectomy, thighlift, backlift, braquio-plasty (for arm flaccidity), mastopexy, and incisional hernia repair. Body contouring procedures can be performed to address the functional and esthetic impairment from skin redundancy more completely following massive weight loss. These can often be accomplished in one stage and are tailored to the individual patient. Body contouring is challenging and requires individualized approaches and intensive follow up.

Unfortunately, in Canada these procedures (with the exception of panniculectomies) are rarely covered by provincial health plans. You should advise patients before surgery about the likelihood of significant skin redundancy and the likely cost of surgical correction. At the time of writing this, the cost ranges between $7,000 and $15,000, depending on the number of different body areas requiring treatment.

[CHAPTER 11: "I CANNOT LOSE WEIGHT!"]

This chapter deals with one of the most difficult patients a physician can face: those who are motivated and claim to be following dietary restrictions and exercising, but who are not achieving weight loss.

Weight loss requires an energy deficit. A weight-stable patient is by definition in a eucaloric state, meaning their caloric intake is roughly equivalent to their caloric expenditure. There are really only three possibilities for a lack of weight loss: the patient is consuming more calories than they believe, they are burning fewer calories than expected, or some combination of the two.

To assess why a patient is not losing weight we need to look at both sides of the energy equation: energy intake and energy output.

ENERGY INTAKE

Patients who are not keeping food diaries or practicing calorie awareness, and those who are not using measuring tools to guide their portions, may still be consuming more calories than they burn despite feeling that they are restricting calories. To assess a patient's calorie awareness, ask them about some of the foods they commonly eat, and about the calories these foods contain. If they are unaware of the correct caloric content, they are clearly not practicing calorie awareness and, given the food environment in which we live, they are almost certainly consuming more calories than they are burning.

These patients would be well advised to begin keeping a food diary and potentially consult with a registered dietitian to learn how to read food labels and understand serving sizes. The aim is not necessarily to count calories (though certainly this would provide the most accurate understanding of intake) but to better understand the caloric content of different food choices.

For most patients, caloric awareness is incredibly eye-opening: a handful of peanuts contains more calories than a large hamburger, the specialty coffee they have every morning has more fat and calories than a piece of deep-fried chicken, and 100% natural fruit juice has more calories drop for drop than sweetened soda.

The most common caloric blind spot is with liquid calories, especially alcohol, juice, and milk. Most patients underestimate or do not even register liquid calories, and liquid portion sizes are also commonly underestimated, especially when alcohol is concerned. We are all more generous than bartenders: one home-poured oversized glass of wine each day can easily add 9 kg (20 lbs) worth of annual wine calories. Combine that with morning glasses of orange juice and skim milk and the annual intake can add up to 18 annual kg (40 annual lbs) of non-satiating liquid calories.

Even moderate consumption of liquid calories can have a very significant impact on daily calorie intake and, in the end, on weight. With all beverages, blind elimination is not the answer. Have the patient decide how much wine, juice, and milk they need in their lives to be happy, and encourage them consume no more and no less than this amount.

> ▸ **Pearl:** One of the most dangerous myths of weight management is that healthy eating can achieve or maintain a healthy weight. Healthy eating and weight management are entirely separate endeavors. The first focuses on the foods we choose to eat; the second on the calories they contain. Many healthy foods are high in calories: consuming one tablespoon of olive oil daily may be a healthy choice, but it adds up to over 5.4 kg (12 lbs) of calories a year.

Food diaries also help identify a patient's eating patterns (including hunger-generating meals and snack skipping). Rendering these accounts more complete and accurate may turn up a great many hidden calories. The patient who says, *"I never eat during the day, I only drink coffee,"* might in fact be adding 960 kcal/day through six large double-doubles at 160 kcal each.

> ▸ **Pearl:** "But I don't eat very much." The energy density of food (calories per gram) may allow a person who does not eat a large volume of food to still consume a great number of calories.

Food diaries also identify where food is being consumed. Restaurant portions and the energy density of restaurant foods have increased dramatically over the years. The result is that even healthy options such as grilled shrimp and citrus salad may have more calories and fat than a fast food burger, fries, and sugared soda.

ENERGY OUTPUT

Lean body mass is the key determinant of resting metabolic rate (RMR), which is respon-sible for 60%–75% of an individual's total daily energy expenditure (TEE). RMR decreases by about 10% from early childhood to adulthood, and another 10% from adulthood to the age of retirement. Factors that directly influence RMR include sympathetic activity, thyroid hormones, genetics, body and/or environmental temperature, and stress. Other factors related to RMR are body surface area, total body weight, lean body mass, gender, age, and aerobic fitness. When metabolically active muscle tissue is lost (as through inactivity, overly rapid weight loss, protein-deficient diets, and chronic disease) and is replaced with metabolically inert depot fat, RMR declines.

Sedentary obese individuals, particularly those who have experienced repeated weight cycling, may have surprisingly low lean body mass and correspondingly low-energy requirements. For example, a 136 kg (300 lb) 50-year-old sedentary female with 50%

lean body mass may have an energy requirement as low as 1500 kcal/day — a low intake by any standards. This woman may report that she eats virtually nothing, but simply cannot lose weight. In order to create an energy deficit of 500 kcal/day and lose 0.5 kg (1 lb)/week, she would have to reduce her caloric intake to around 1000 kcal per day, an amount that would almost certainly not be enjoyable for the patient or sustainable over the long run. This patient would almost certainly require either pharmacotherapy or surgery to sustain weight loss.

▸ **Pearl:** To estimate TEE, use the Mifflin St-Jeor equations reproduced below (or type "Calorie calculator" into an Internet search engine and save yourself the math). For a 0.5 kg (1 lb) per week weight loss, a patient needs to consume roughly 500 kcal less than their TEE per day.

Male TEE = [10×wt (kg) + 6.25×ht (cm) – 5×age + 5] x AQ

Female TEE = [10×wt (kg) + 6.25×ht (cm) – 5×age – 161] x AQ

Activity Quotient (AQ)

1.200 = sedentary (little or no exercise)

1.375 = lightly active (light exercise/sports 1–3 days/week)

1.550 = moderately active (moderate exercise/sports 3–5 days/week)

1.725 = very active (hard exercise/sports 6–7 days a week)

1.900 = extra active (very hard exercise/sports and physical job)

For most patients, exercise contributes only minimally to TEE. Modern life does not leave much time for exercise, and most jobs are anything but physical. Even in occupations that still involve generous amounts of physical activity (e.g., waiter, construction worker, landscaper, etc.) total activity-related energy expenditure may only be in the neighbourhood of 1200–1500 kcal — the equivalent of one fast food value meal and a specialty coffee.

The tendency among patients and physicians to grossly overestimate the calories burned through exercise puts patients who initiate an exercise program at risk for actually gaining weight unless they remain acutely calorie aware. They tend to overcompensate for exercise by consuming more extra calories than they burn.

While we do not advocate that you encourage your patients to take on more exercise than they can actually enjoy (as this will likely lead to a short-lived exercise program), many health professionals and governments are now recommending that patients try to take 10,000 steps a day. To give your patients some perspective, the following chart compares the estimated calories burned through 1.5 to 2 hours of daily walking, which is (roughly how long the recommended 10,000 steps would take) to the calories contained in some commonly consumed foods:

Weight		Calories		
45 – 54 kg	(100 – 119 lbs.)	420		
54.5 – 63 kg	(120 – 139 lbs.)	440		
63.5 – 72 kg	(140 – 159 lbs.)	460		
72.5 – 81 kg	(160 – 179 lbs.)	480		
81.5 – 90 kg	(180 – 199 lbs.)	500		
90.5 – 99 kg	(200 – 219 lbs.)	520		
99.5 – 108 kg	(220 – 239 lbs.)	540		
108.5 – 117 kg	(240 – 259 lbs.)	560		
117.5 – 131 kg	(260 – 289 lbs.)	580		

Food	Calories	Steps	Time
Big pop (900 mL or 32 oz)	373	7,500	1.0 hr.
Garden vegetable sandwich	450	9,000	1.5 hr.
Regular fast food meal	790	16,000	2.2 hr.
Supersized fast food meal	1100	21,000	3.0 hr.

▸ **Pearl:** Exercise for weight management is cumulative rather than consecutive, and studies suggest that obtaining >250 minutes weekly greatly increases a person's likelihood of maintaining a weight loss.

"I'VE HIT A PLATEAU"

Is there really such a thing as a weight-loss plateau? Is it physiologically possible for a patient to have a daily caloric deficit one week and none the next? More often than not, the patient is simply consuming more calories than they believe, either through restaurant meals, unmeasured portions, or faulty caloric assumptions. Alternatively, the scale may be weighing something else. Scales are not especially sensitive in the short term, as they will measure constipation, clothing, and level of hydration — daily fluid shifts in morbidly obese patients can exceed 5 kg (10 lbs). Therefore, a patient who has been sustaining a caloric deficit may in fact be losing true weight while the scale remains unchanged or even shows weight gain. The good news for such patients is that the scale eventually catches up to their efforts.

It is also important to know that as patients become smaller, so do their resting energy expenditures. Every part of our bodies burns calories, so the less body there is, the fewer calories that are burned. While this decrease in REE can be offset somewhat by regular exercise, if patients lose enough weight, they will be burning fewer daily calories.

While by no means a true mathematical model, the easiest way to explain this phenomenon to patients is to tell them that for every percentage point of their bodies they lose, they will likely burn 1% fewer calories. Therefore, if they want to permanently lose 10% of their weight, they will need to find enjoyable ways of living on 10% fewer calories.

▸ **Pearl:** To determine if a patient has reached a "plateau" or an actual weight-loss floor, you need only ask them two questions:

1. Could you eat any fewer calories and still enjoy your life?
2. Could you exercise any more and still enjoy your life?

If the answer to either question is "Yes," then they have reached a "plateau." If the answer to both questions is "No" and their weight has not change in 6-8 weeks, then they have reached a floor where no further weight loss is likely to occur.

[CHAPTER 12: AFTER WEIGHT LOSS]

Dramatic weight loss, particularly for patients who conquer morbid or super-morbid obesity, brings substantial emotional and physical challenges as patients contend with changes in their body images, identity, and lifestyle. This is true regardless of the methods employed to lose weight. As weight loss becomes apparent to others, patients will experience a change in attitude from partners, family, co-workers, and even complete strangers. While most patients will experience this as positive, increased attention from others can pose a substantial emotional challenge for patients who are uncomfortable dealing with this new attention.

Interestingly, many friends and co-workers may respond negatively to ongoing weight loss, and respond with statements like, "You should stop losing weight, you don't look well," even when the patient still carries enough weight to present serious medical risk. This type of comment may have roots in evolutionary biology or experiential observations that have taught us to recognize weight loss as a consequence of serious illness. Anecdotally, this type of negative reaction tends to coincide with the 15%–20% weight-loss mark, and it may be helpful for you to forewarn patients that they might expect such comments. Whether positive or negative, increased attention can sometimes result in aggression, anxiety, fear, and frustration, and may give rise to new social phobias, partnership problems, spousal jealousy, unwanted sexual interest, and/or abuse.

Clinicians must be aware that dramatic weight loss can have real negative consequences and ensure that patients know they are available for ongoing support and counselling.

APPENDIX A:
COMMERCIAL WEIGHT-LOSS PROGRAMS

Many clinicians are pressed for time, and therefore may encourage their patients to seek out additional help for their weight-management efforts. Consequently, we feel it is essential that physicians make themselves aware of the resources that their patients may choose to use. While by no means an exhaustive list, here are some of the more common approaches your patients may take to find weight-loss advice.

Diet Books
At the time of writing, there were more than 52,000 different diet books available on Amazon.com. All of them work — that is, so long as calories consumed are less than calories burned. Unfortunately, as far as long-term success goes, there is at least a 95% failure rate for most diets.

For the most part, diet books can be divided into three categories: *Low-fat, Low-carb* and *Desperate. Low-fat* aims for fat intake to reflect less than 20% of daily calories. *Low-carb* aims for carbohydrate intake to reflect less than 40% of daily calories. Desperate simply looks for miracles.

Diets fail due to restricting foods to the point of hunger or suffering. Regardless of how much weight is lost, eventually patients choose to stop suffering. Then, of course, old habits (along with old calories and old weight) return.

Government Diet Recommendations
Neither the American Food Pyramid nor Canada's Food Guide to Healthy Eating were designed with weight management in mind. Following either while ignoring calories could easily lead patients with healthy weight to gain weight, and overweight patients not to lose it.

Commercial Weight-Loss Programs
A myriad of commercial weight-loss programs is available. It is important for physicians to be aware of what they entail, and to help their patients choose wisely.

The 10 Checks of a Healthy Weight-Loss Program
Unfortunately, not everyone involved in weight management uses evidence-based practices. Fraud, either well-intentioned but misinformed or overtly unethical, runs rampant in the weight-loss industry.

To help your patients navigate through the unregulated maze of commercial weight-loss options, feel free to photocopy the following check list. Simply advise your patients that unless all boxes are checked, they should not enroll in the program.

• The program is not a one-size-fits-all diet and has individualized nutritional, exercise and behavioural components.

- Nutritional advice is provided by a physician or a registered dietitian.*

- Exercise is encouraged but physical activity is promoted at a gradual, rather than at an injury-inducing rapid pace.

- Reasonable weight-loss goals are set at a pace of 3 lb per week at most, and the program does not promise or imply dramatic, rapid, weight loss as an outcome.

- The program does not require the outlay of large sums of money at the start or make clients sign contracts for expensive, long-term programs without the option of at least partial refunds (which you should discuss before enrolling).

- The program does not promote diets <800 kcal daily, and if diets contain <1200 kcal daily, they are supervised by a physician.

- The program does not require the use or purchase of any products, supplements, vitamins, or injections.

- The program does not make outlandish claims such as, "You will only lose fat," or, "We can target problem areas".

- The program has an established maintenance program available.

- The program provides you with statistics that include the percentage of clients who drop out, the average percentage of weight clients lose, and the average weight loss sustained following completion of their maintenance program.

*Note: Outside of Quebec, the term "nutritionist" is not protected by law in Canada and therefore we cannot consider someone who refers to themselves as a "nutritionist" to be a reliable and trusted source of information.

The Best Diet
Your patient's best diet has fewer calories than their current diet and satisfies hunger while retaining livability. In the history of medicine, one diet has never been proven to be better than another for weight loss, and especially for long-term weight-loss maintenance.

The Bottom Line
Patients must be able to confidently say they can live with their choices for the rest of their lives, or weight will return.

[APPENDIX B: FOOD DIARY]

Please feel free to copy this simple, sample food diary (next page) and provide it to your patients.

The diary is very simple to use. It has one column for time, ample space for what was eaten, a column to indicate whether or not the amount was physically measured (spoons, cups, grams, etc.), a column for calories, and an optional column for people with diabetes who wish to track their carbohyrates.

At the bottom of the page is space to indicate what activities a patient undertook, their daily step count, and minutes of exercise.

MEASURED	DATE:	TIME	CALORIES	CARBS
	BREAKFAST			
	SNACK			
	LUNCH			
	SNACK			
	DINNER			
	SNACK			
	TOTALS			

STEPS TAKEN:	
MINUTES OF EXERCISE:	

[APPENDIX C: SOME SNACKING IDEAS]

For many patients, the most foreign suggestion you will make is that they eat frequently, even if they are not responding to an internal hunger cue. Consequently, most patients are not accustomed to snacking and often struggle with snack ideas, especially snacks that include protein. The following list offers some easy suggestions for snacks that contain protein:

- 2 Tbsp peanut butter and crackers
- Cottage cheese and fruit
- 1 oz cheese and crackers
- 1/2 turkey sandwich
- Boiled egg and pita
- 1 oz cheese and fruit
- Cottage cheese and veggies
- Prepackaged 1 oz bags of nuts (keep them in your car, purse or desk at work)
- 1/2 peanut butter sandwich
- Flavoured tuna and crackers
- 1/3 cup hummus and pita
- Boiled egg, salsa and crackers
- 1/2 cup Cereal and 1/2 oz nuts
- Leftover dinner
- 1 oz nuts and 1–2 cups popcorn
- Yogurt and 1 oz nuts
- Cheese strings, Baby Bell or Laughing Cow cheese
- Grains First crackers by Dare
- Ryvita crackers
- Individual cottage cheese cups

[PERMISSIONS]

Page 8 – **Table 1: What's in a name?** Reprinted with permission from Macmillan Publishers Ltd: (Wadden T., Didie, E. What's in a Name? Patients' Preferred Terms for Describing Obesity. *Obesity Research* 11; 1140–1146: 2003.

Page 11 – **Table 2: Prochaska's Readiness for Change model.** Adapted with permission from American Psychological Association: Prochaska, J.O. *et al.* In Search of How People Change: Applications to Addictive Behaviors. *American Psychologist* 47, 9; 1102–1114: 1992.

Page 18 – **Table 3: Average weight gain with selected novel antipsychotics.** Adapted from Wetterling, T. Body weight gain with atypical antipsychotics. A comparative review. *Drug Safety* 24; 59–73: 2001.

Page 24 – **Table 4: Diagnosis of binge-eating disorder.** Adapted with permission from Macmillan Publishers Ltd: *Obesity Research* (Tanosky-Kraff, *et al.* Eating disorder or disordered eating? Nonnormative eating patterns in obese individuals. *Obesity Research* 12; 1361–1366: 2004.

Page 28 – **Table 5. Antipsychotics and potential for weight gain.** Adapted with permission from American Psychiatric Publishing, Inc.: Allison., David, B. *et al.* Antipsychotic-Induced Weight Gain: A Comprehensive Research Synthesis. *American Journal of Psychiatry* 156, 11; 1686–1696: 1999.

Page 37 – **List of eating pattern criteria.** Adapted with permission from Macmillan Publishers Ltd: *Obesity Research* (Tanosky-Kraff, *et al.* Eating disorder or disordered eating? Nonnormative eating patterns in obese individuals. *Obesity Research* 12; 1361–1366: 2004.

Page 43 – **Table 7: Waist circumference as measure of central obesity (pragmatic cut-offs).** Reprinted with permission from Elsevier: Alberti, K.G.M.M. et al., The metabolic syndrome – a new worldwide definition. *The Lancet* 366; 1059–1062: c 2005.

Page 68 – **Table 8: Revised diagnostic criteria for serotonin syndrome.** Reprinted with permission from the *Canadian Medical Association Journal:* (Birmes, P. *et al.* Serotonin syndrome: a brief review. *Canadian Medical Association Journal* 168, 11; 1439–1442: 2003.

Page 70 – **Table 9: Comparison of various features of the anti-obesity drugs orlistat and sibutramine.** Adapted with permission from Wolters Kluwer Pharma Solutions: Better than slim chances for orlistat and sibutramine to promote weight loss. *Drugs & Therapy Perspectives* 15 (12) 1–6 (19 June 2000).

Page 77 – **List of non-fatal complications from surgery.** Adapted from Abell, Minocha. Gastrointestinal complications of bariatric surgery: Diagnosis and therapy. *American Journal of Medical Sciences* 331: 4; 214–218: (2006).

[INDEX]

[INDEX]

[INDEX]

[INDEX]

[INDEX]

CPSIA information can be obtained at www.ICGtesting.com
235220LV00002B/37/P